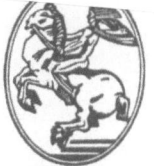

ACTA NEUROCHIRURGICA
SUPPLEMENTUM 25

Glossary
of Neurotraumatology

About 200 Neurotraumatological Terms
and Their Definitions
in English, German, Spanish, and French

Edited by
E. S. Gurdjian, J. Brihaye, J. C. Christensen,
R. A. Frowein, S. Lindgren, W. Luyendijk,
G. Norlén, A. K. Ommaya, I. Oprescu,
A. de Vasconcellos Marques, R. P. Vigouroux

SPRINGER-VERLAG
WIEN   NEW YORK

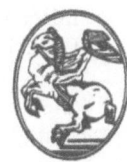

Library of Congress Cataloging in Publication Data. Main entry under title: Glossary of neurotraumatology. (Acta neurochirurgica: Supplementum; 25) English, French, German, and Spanish. 1. Nervous system-Wounds and injuries-Dictionaries-Polyglot. 2. Dictionaries, Polyglot. I. Gurdjian, Elisha Stephen, 1900-   . II. Series. RD593.G56. 617'.1. 78-15626.

ISBN-13:978-3-211-81481-9   e-ISBN-13:978-3-7091-8515-5

DOI: 10.1007/978-3-7091-8515-5

Preface

The Committee of Neurotraumatology of the World Federation of Neurosurgical Societies decided to elaborate a Glossary of Neurotraumatology, and for this purpose appointed a subgroup of members of this Committee, headed by Dr. E. S. Gurdjian, whose report follows this preface.

The main reason for the Committee's decision was the hope that the diffusion of the Glossary through "Acta Neurochirurgica" may bring about a better understanding of neurotraumatological terminology on a worldwide scale. The Glossary should facilitate the classification and the comparison of traumatic lesions of the Nervous System. It will consequently be easier to compile statistics and correctly interpret the informations thus obtained.

The very commendable initiative of the Congress of Neurological Surgeons in revising the terminology of head injuries and in publishing this work in Vol. 12 (1966) of "Clinical Neurosurgery" constitutes an important contribution. In 1977 the Glossary now presented endeavours to complete and bring up to date the definitions of anatomical or physiological modifications in the neurotraumatological field.

We wish to express our thanks to Dr. Gurdjian and to the other members of the Neurotraumatological Committee who were responsible for the elaboration of this Glossary and whose efforts to standardise, as much as possible, the language used by scientists of different nationalities, have resulted in a better understanding between neurosurgeons.

After the adoption of English as the universal neurosurgical language, the initiative to standardise neurotraumatological definitions should be understood, and the opportunity it offers taken by all those connected with such an important sector of Neurosurgery. Furthermore, its translation into three other languages will undoubtedly be an added advantage, since the Glossary should have as far reaching a diffusion as possible.

And thus, we hope, the purpose of the Neurotraumatological Committee when it undertook to elaborate this Glossary will have been accomplished.

Dr. A. de Vasconcellos Marques,
Chairman of the Committee of Neurotraumatology
of the World Federation of Neurosurgical Societies

The Report of the Committee on Terminology in Neurotraumatology (Glossary) of the World Federation of Neurosurgical Societies

The Committee of Terminology in Neurotraumatology has prepared a Glossary of Neurotraumatology. The work was accomplished by correspondence and meetings of the committee one day in Oxford, October, 1975; three days in Brussels in October, 1976; and two days in São Paulo in June, 1977. The French translation was prepared by Drs. Brihaye and Vigouroux, the German translation by Dr. Frowein, and the Spanish by Dr. Christensen.

We received much help and suggestions from Drs. Pevehouse, Voris, and Walker. The head injury nomenclature prepared by a Committee of the Congress of Neurological Surgeons and published in Clinical Neurosurgery, Volume 12, 1966, was also freely used. The term "traumatic unconsciousness" was discussed in detail, but clouding of the conscious state after trauma was left for consideration in the future.

The committee thanks the editors and the publishers of "Acta Neurochirurgica" for publishing the Glossary.

October 1978

The Editors

Gurdjian, Elisha Stephen, emer. Prof. Neurosurgery, Wayne State University; Suite 808 Professional Plaza, 3800 Woodward Avenue, Detroit, MI 48201, U.S.A.

Brihaye, Jean, Prof., Directeur de la Clinique Neurochirurgicale, Université Libre de Bruxelles, rue Héger-Bordet, 1, B-1000 Bruxelles, Belgium.

Christensen, Juan Carlos, Assist. Prof., Universidad de Buenos Aires; Hospital Francés de Buenos Aires; Hospital Británico de Buenos Aires; Ayacucho 2151, 4° P., RA-1112 Buenos Aires, Argentina.

Frowein, Reinhold Alexander, Prof., Direktor der Neurochirurgischen Universitätsklinik, Joseph-Stelzmann-Straße 9, D-5000 Köln 41, Federal Republic of Germany.

Lindgren, Sten, Prof., Göteborgs Universitet; Sahlgrenska Sjukhuset, S-413 45 Göteborg, Sweden.

Luyendijk, Willem, Prof., Rijksuniversiteit te Leiden; Academisch Ziekenhuis, Rijnsburgerweg 10, Leiden, The Netherlands.

Norlén, Gösta, Prof. emer., Linnégatan 35, S-114 47 Stockholm, Sweden.

Ommaya, Ayub Khan, Acting Chief, Surgical Neurology Branch, National Institute of Neurological and Communicative Disorders and Stroke, National Institutes of Health, Bethesda, MD 20014, U.S.A.

Oprescu, Ion, Chief Neurosurgeon, Neurosurgical Clinic, 25, C. A. Rosetti, Bucureşti, I., Romania.

Vasconcellos Marques, António de, Director do Serviço de Neurocirurgia, Hospitais Civis de Lisboa, Rua do Prior, 22, Lisboa, Portugal.

Vigouroux, Robert Paul, Prof., Université d'Aix-Marseille; C. H. U. Timone, 264, Rue Saint-Pierre, F-13385 Marseille, Cedex 4, France.

Glossary of Neurotraumatology

Neurotraumatologisches Wörterbuch

Glosario de Neurotraumatología

Glossaire de Neurotraumatologie

1

Abscess: Collection of pus within tissues (see also *empyema*).

Abszeß: Eiteransammlung in einer nicht vorgebildeten, allseitig abgeschlossenen Höhlenbildung eines Gewebes (siehe auch *empyema*).

Acute anterior cervical cord syndrome: see *syndrome*, acute anterior cervical syndrome.

Akutes zervikales Spinalis-Anterior-Syndrom: (siehe *syndrome*, acute anterior cervical syndrome).

Acute central cervical cord syndrome: see *syndrome*, acute central cervical cord.

Akute zentrale Halsmarkschädigung: (siehe *syndrome*, acute central cervical cord).

Amnesia post-traumatic: loss of memory for events before the injury—retrograde amnesia; loss of memory of events after the injury—anterograde amnesia.

Amnesie, posttraumatische: Erinnerungslücke; retrograd: für Ereignisse vor dem Unfall; anterograd: für Ereignisse nach dem Unfall.

Anastomosis, nerve: see *neurorrhaphy*.

Anastomose, Nerven-: siehe *neurorrhaphy*.

Aneurysm, dissecting: splitting or dissection of an arterial wall by blood entering through an intimal tear or by interstitial hemorrhage, usually spontaneous, occasionnally traumatic.

Aneurysma dissecans (intramurales A.): Auftreibung einer Arterienwand infolge Eindringens von Blut zwischen einzelne Wandschichten durch Einriß der Intima oder interstitielle Blutung, gewöhnlich spontan, gelegentlich traumatisch.

Aneurysm, false, traumatic: pulsating encapsulated hematoma in communication with a traumatic ruptured artery.

Aneurysma, falsches, traumatisches (Aneurysma spurium): pulsierendes, abgekapseltes Hämatom, das mit einer Arterien-Verletzung in offener Verbindung steht.

Absceso: Colección de pus dentro de un tejido (ver también *empiema*).

Abcès : collection de pus à l'intérieur d'un tissu (voir aussi *empyème*).

ver: *síndrome agudo anterior de la médula cervical.*

Syndrome médullaire cervical antérieur aigu : (voir ce terme) (ou *syndrome antéro-médullaire aigu*).

ver: *síndrome agudo central de la médula cervical.*

Syndrome médullaire cervical central aigu : (voir ce terme) (ou *syndrome cervical-centro-médullaire aigu*).

Amnesia post-traumática: la pérdida de memoria para los hechos previos al accidente se llama amnesia retrógrada; aquella para los hechos posteriores al accidente se llama anterógrada.

Amnésie post-traumatique : perte de mémoire des événements précédant l'accident : amnésie rétrograde ; perte de mémoire des événements postérieurs à l'accident : amnésie antérograde.

Anastomosis, nervio: ver *neurorrafia*.

Anastomose nerveuse : voir *neurorraphie*.

Aneurisma disecante: separación de las capas de la pared arterial provocada por la entrada de sangre a través de un desgarro de la intima o por hemorragia intersticial. Generalmente de origen espontáneo pero ocasionalmente traumático.

Anévrysme disséquant (dissection artérielle) : clivage ou dissection de la paroi artérielle par du sang pénétrant par une plaie de l'intima ou par une hémorragie interstitielle, généralement spontanée, parfois traumatique.

Aneurisma, falso, traumático: hematoma pulsátil y encapsulado en communicación con una arteria rota por trauma.

Faux anévrysme traumatique : hématome encapsulé et pulsatile en communication avec une rupture artérielle.

1*

Aneurysm, true, spontaneous, traumatic: localized dilatation of an artery resulting from partial disruption of its wall.

Arachnitis: see *arachnoiditis.*

Arachnoiditis: inflammatory reaction of the pia and arachnoid (see also *meningitis*, traumatic).

Arachnoiditis, adhesive: *(leptomeningeal* Fibrosis): thickening of the leptomeninges, associated with varying degrees of obliteration of the sub-arachnoid space.

Arteriovenous communication: craniocerebral-spinal, traumatic: communication between craniocerebral or spinal arteries and veins due to trauma.

Atlantoaxial dislocation: dislocation between the atlas and axis.

Atrophy, post-traumatic, brain: loss of brain substance, local or diffuse, following trauma.

Automatism, post-traumatic immediate: a post-traumatic state in which the patient performs automatically without immediate or late memory of his behavior.

Aneurysma, wahres, spontanes, traumatisches: echtes Aneurysma: umschriebene (sackförmige) Ausweitung einer Arterie infolge umschriebener Ausbuchtung aller ihrer Wandschichten.

Arachnitis: siehe *arachnoiditis.*

Arachn(oid)itis: entzündliche Reaktion der Pia und Arachnoidea (siehe auch *meningitis* traumatic).

Arachn(oid)itis, adhaesive: Verdickung der weichen Hirnhäute, verbunden mit verschiedengradiger Obliteration des Subarachnoidalraumes.

Arteriovenöses Aneurysma: traumatischer arteriovenöser Kurzschluß zerebraler oder spinaler Arterien und Venen infolge einer Verletzung.

Atlanto-axiale Luxation: Luxation zwischen Atlas und Epistropheus.

Atrophie, posttraumatische, Hirn-: umschriebener oder allgemeiner Hirnsubstanz-Verlust nach einem Hirntrauma.

Automatismen, unmittelbare, posttraumatische: automatenhafte Bewegungen im akuten posttraumatischen Stadium, ohne daß an dieses Verhalten unmittelbar oder später eine Erinnerung besteht.

Aneurisma verdadero (espontáneo, traumático): dilatación localizada de una arteria como resultado de una alteración parcial de su pared.

Anévrysme spontané ou traumatique : dilatation localisée d'une artère consécutive à la rupture partielle de sa paroi.

Arachnitis: ver *aracnoiditis.*

Arachnitis : voir *arachnoïdite.*

Aracnoiditis: reacción inflamatoria de la pia-aracnoides (ver también *Meningitis* traumática).

Arachnoïdite : réaction inflammatoire de la pie-mère et de l'arachnoïde (voir aussi *méningite posttraumatique*).

Aracnoiditis adhesiva (leptomeningitis fibrosa): engrosamiento de las leptomeninges, asociado a veces con un grado variable de obliteración de los espacios subaracnoideos.

Arachnoïdite adhésive (fibrose leptoméningée) : épaississement de la leptoméninge, associée à des degrés variés de cloisonnement des espaces sous-arachnoidiens.

Comunicación arteriovenosa, craneocerebral-espinal, traumática: communicación entre arterias y venas craniocerebrales o espinales por trauma.

Fistule artérioveineuse craniocérébrale, spinale (rachidienne) traumatique : fistule entre une artère cranio-cérébrale ou spinale et une veine, consécutive au traumatisme.

Dislocación atlando-axoidea: Dislocación entre el atlas y la odontoides.

Dislocation atlantoïdo-axoïdienne : dislocation entre l'atlas et l'axis.

Atrofia cerebral post-traumática: pérdida de substancia cerebral, localizada o difusa, consecutiva a un trauma.

Atrophie cérébrale post-traumatique : diminution de volume du cerveau, localisée ou diffuse, consécutive au traumatisme.

Automatismo post-traumático inmediato: estado post-traumático en el cual el paciente actúa automáticamente sin recuerdo inmediato o alejado de su comportamiento.

Automatisme post-traumatique, immédiat : un état suivant immédiatement un traumatisme et au cours duquel le sujet agit selon un mode automatique sans souvenir immédiat ou ultérieur de son comportement.

Axonotmesis: degeneration of the endoneural sheath with marked axonal discontinuity, with loss of conduction until the axon has regenerated (Grade II); (see also *neuropraxia* and *neurotmesis*).

Axonotmesis: (Nervenverletzung Grad II) traumatische Kontinuitätsunterbrechung der Axone mit Wallerscher Degeneration des Endoneuriums aber erhaltenem Endoneuralrohr; bis zur Regeneration der Axone ist die Nervenleitfähigkeit aufgehoben (siehe auch *neuropraxia* und *neurotmesis*).

Brace, spine: an apparatus to immobilize all or part of the spine (see also *splint*).

Stützkorsett: Gerät zur Ruhigstellung eines Teiles oder der ganzen Wirbelsäule (siehe auch *splint*).

Brain death: total irreversible loss of brain function.

Hirn-Tod: irreversibles Aussetzen aller Hirnfunktionen.

Brain injury: closed, open (see brain injury, closed, open) in *craniocerebral injury*.

Hirnverletzung, geschlossen — offen: (siehe brain injury, closed-open in *craniocerebral injury*).

Brain syndrome, traumatic chronic: see *encephalopathy*, traumatic chronic.

Posttraumatisches, hirnorganisches Syndrom: langanhaltende posttraumatische Hirnfunktionsstörung (siehe *encephalopathy*, traumatic chronic).

Caput succedaneum: circumscribed area of scalp edema caused by pressure on the scalp in the birth canal.

Geburtsgeschwulst: umschriebenes Ödem der Kopfhaut infolge Druckwirkung im Geburtskanal.

Carpal tunnel syndrome: see *syndrome*, carpal tunnel.

Carpaltunnel-Syndrom: siehe *syndrome*, carpal tunnel).

Axonotmesis: degeneración de las vainas endoneurales con marcada discontinuidad axónica y pérdida de la conducción nerviosa hasta que se haya regenerado el axón (grado II) (ver también *neuropraxia* y *neurotmesis*).

Axonotmésis : dégénérescence de la gaine endoneurale avec rupture d'axones, responsable d'une perte de conduction nerveuse tant que les axones n'ont pas régénéré (stade II) (voir aussi *neuropraxie et neurotmesis*).

Ortesis espinal: aparato para inmovilizar la columna vertebral en su totalidad o en parte (también minerva o corset).

Corset, minerve : appareil qui sert à immobiliser la colonne rachidienne. Le terme corset est utilisé pour le rachis lombaire et dorsal, le terme minerve pour le rachis cervical. L'association des deux, permet une immobilisation totale du rachis.

Muerte cerebral: pérdida irreversible y total de la función cerebral.

Mort cérébrale : disparition irréversible des fonctions cérébrales.

Trauma cerebral, cerrado-abierto: ver *trauma encefalo-craneano*.

Traumatisme cérébral : voir traumatisme cérébral dans la rubrique: *traumatismes cranio-cérébraux*.

Sindrome cerebral crónico de origen traumático: ver *encefalopatia crónica traumática*.

Encéphalopathie chronique post-traumatique : voir ce terme.

Caput succedaneum: edema circunscripto del cuero cabelludo causado por presión de las paredes del canal del parto sobre la cabeza del niño.

Caput succedaneum : oedème du cuir chevelu dû à une compression lors de l'accouchement.

Carpal tunnel syndrome: ver *sindrome* del túnel carpiano.

Syndrome du canal carpien : voir ce terme.

Cauliflower ear (Boxer's ear): thickening and induration of the ear with distorsion of contours following extravasation of blood within its tissues.

Blumenkohlohr, Boxer Ohr: Verdickung und Verhärtung des Ohres mit verstrichenen Konturen infolge Blutaustritt in das Gewebe.

Causalgia: persistent burning pain generally in the distribution of an injured nerve and usually accompanied with autonomic disturbances.

Kausalgie: anhaltender, brennender Schmerz, gewöhnlich im Versorgungsgebiet eines verletzten Nervs und meist verbunden mit vegetativen Störungen.

Causalgia, major: severe causalgia, especially in the distribution of the median or sciatic nerves.

Kausalgie, schwere: besonders im Versorgungsgebiet des Nervus medianus und Nervus ischiadicus.

Causalgia, minor: less severe causalgia associated with laceration or bruise of a limb.

Kausalgie, leichte: bei Verletzung oder Quetschung eines Gliedes.

Craniocerebral injury: injury of the brain and its coverings.

Schädel-Hirn-Trauma: mehr oder weniger starke Beteiligung des Hirns im Rahmen der Schädelverletzung.

Craniocerebral injury, brain injury, closed: no fracture of the skull; skin and/or mucous membranes may be lacerated, but dura-mater is intact.

Schädel-Hirn-Trauma, Gedeckte Hirnverletzung: Haut und/oder Mukosa und/oder Schädelknochen können verletzt sein, die Dura aber ist intakt.

Oreja en coliflor (oreja de boxeador): engrosamiento e induración de la oreja y deformación de sus bordes como consecuencia de extravasación sanguínea en sus tejidos.

Oreille en chou-fleur (oreille de boxeur) : cette expression populaire n'est pas utilisée en terminologie médicale : épaississement et induration de l'oreille avec distorsion de ses contours consécutifs à une extravasation de sang dans les tissus du pavillon de l'oreille.

Causalgia: dolor quemante y persistente, por lo común en el territorio de un nervio lesionado, que suele acompañarse de alteraciones del sistema nervioso autónomo.

Causalgie : douleur persistante à type de brûlure siégeant généralement dans le territoire d'un nerf traumatisé et généralement accompagnée de perturbations neuro-végétatives.

Causalgia mayor: causalgia severa, especialmente en el territorio de los nervios mediano o ciático.

Causalgie majeure : causalgie violente, siégeant particulièrement dans le territoire du médian et du sciatique.

Causalgia menor: causalgia leve, asociada a laceración o contusión de un miembro.

Causalgie mineure : causalgie moins violente, associée à une contusion plus ou moins importante ou à l' écrasement d'un menbre.

Trauma encefalocraneano: lesión del cerebro y sus envolturas.

Traumatisme craniocérébral : traumatisme du cerveau et de ses enveloppes.

Trauma encefalocraneano, trauma encefálico cerrado: no hay fractura de cráneo. La piel y/o las membranas mucosas pueden estar laceradas pero la duramadre está intacta.

Traumatisme craniocérébral: traumatisme cérébral fermé : il n'y a pas de fracture du crâne. Il peut exister une plaie des enveloppes cutanées et/ou des membranes muqueuses, mais la dure-mère est intacte.

Craniocerebral injury, brain injury, open: skin and/or mucous membranes and dura-mater are lacerated with fracture of the skull in the same area.

Schädel-Hirn-Trauma, Offene Hirnverletzung: Haut und/oder Mukosa-Verletzung, Fraktur *und Dura-Verletzung* in der gleichen Region.

Craniocerebral injury, skull fracture, closed: fracture of the skull, but skin, mucous membranes and dura-mater are intact.

Schädelfraktur, geschlossene: ohne Verletzung der Haut und/ oder der Mukosa sowie Dura.

Craniocerebral injury, skull fracture, open: fracture of skull, skin and/or mucous membranes are lacerated, but dura-mater is intact.

Schädelfraktur, offene: mit darüberliegender Haut und/oder Schleimhautverletzung, aber die Dura darunter ist intakt.

Cephalhematoma: collection of blood beneath the pericranium.

Kephalhämatom, Kopfblutgeschwulst: subperiostales Hämatom, z. B. bei Neugeborenen.

Cerebritis (encephalitis): inflammation of the brain which may or may not lead to suppuration.

Enzephalitis: Entzündung des Gehirns mit oder ohne eitriger Einschmelzung.

Cervical myospasm: see *syndrome*, neck, post-traumatic.

Zervikaler Muskelhartspann, Myogelosen: siehe *syndrome*, neck, post-traumatic.

Cervical tension syndrome: see *syndrome*, neck, post-traumatic.

Nackensteife: siehe *syndrome*, neck, post-traumatic.

Trauma encefalocraneano, trauma encefálico abierto: la piel y/o las membranas mucosas y la duramadre están laceradas y hay fractura de cráneo en la misma zona.

Traumatisme craniocérébral: traumatisme cérébral ouvert : il existe une plaie des enveloppes cutanées et/ou des membranes muqueuses, ainsi que de la dure-mère, avec fracture du crâne dans la même région.

Trauma encefalocraneano, trauma craneano, cerrado: fractura de craneo pero la piel, las mucosas y la dura están intactas.

Traumatisme craniocérébral: traumatisme cranien fermé : il y a une fracture du crâne, mais les enveloppes cutanées les membranes muqueuses et la dure-mère sont intactes.

Trauma encefalocraneano, trauma craneano, abierto: fractura de cráneo. Piel y/o mucosas laceradas pero la duramadre está sana.

Traumatisme craniocérébral: traumatisme crânien ouvert : il y a une fracture du crâne et une plaie des enveloppes cutanées et/ou des membranes muqueuses, mais la dure-mère est intacte.

Cefalohematoma: colección sanguínea bajo el pericráneo.

Céphalhématome : collection de sang sous le péricrâne.

Cerebritis (encefalitis): inflamación del cerebro que puede evolucionar o nó hacia la supuración.

Encéphalite : voir ce terme.

Espasmo muscular cervical: ver *síndrome cervical post-traumático.*

Contracture des muscles cervicaux (terme peu usité) : voir *syndrome cervical post-traumatique.*

Síndrome de tensión cervical: ver *síndrome cervical post-traumático.*

Syndrome de tension cervicale (terme non usité) : voir *syndrome cervical post-traumatique.*

Chin sling: a bandage with a longitudinal opening passed over the head and neck. It may be positioned in a manner to support the chin and the back of the head and neck for traction of the neck and immobilization (see also *traction*, halter).

Kinn-Schleuder: Zug-Vorrichtung mit Longitudinal-Öffnungs-Vorrichtung, um über Kopf und Nacken zu gehen. Sie muß so an Kinn und Nacken-Hinterkopf angelegt werden, daß sie eine Extension und Ruhigstellung des Nackens bewirkt (siehe auch *traction*, halter).

Cicatrix, brain: a lesion resulting from repair of brain injury characterized by proliferation of mesodermal and ectodermal (glial) elements.

Hirnnarbe: Defekt-Zustand nach umschriebener Hirnverletzung, charakterisiert durch Proliferation mesodermaler und gliöser Elemente.

Cicatrix (scar), meningocerebral: scarring and adhesions involving contiguous brain and meninges.

Narbe, Hirn-: Narbenbildung der Hirnsubstanz und Verklebung mit den Hirnhäuten.

Coma: syndrome of unconsciousness (see *unconsciousness*) plus, more or less, neurological and autonomic disturbances. The degree of severity is related to incidence and duration of the disturbances.

Coma: Syndrom mit Bewußtlosigkeit und mehr oder weniger ausgeprägten neurologischen und vegetativen Funktionsstörungen. Der Schweregrad des Comas steht in Relation zum Auftreten und zur Dauer dieser Störungen.

Compression fracture: see *fracture*, compression.

Kompressionsfraktur: siehe *fracture*, compression.

Compression nerve, paralysis: see *paralysis*, compression nerve.

Nerven-Drucklähmung, Nerven-Kompression: siehe *paralysis*, compression nerve.

Fronda mentoniana: vendaje con apertura longitudinal para el cuello que sirve para traccionar la cabeza. Puede colocarse de manera que apoyen el mentón y la nuca para la tracción e inmovilización cervical.

Fronde : bandage en tissu avec un chef sous-mentonnier et un chef sous-occipital, utilisé pour réaliser une traction et une immobilisation du rachis cervical (voir aussi *traction,* extension).

Cicatriz cerebral: alteración estructural secuelar de una lesión cerebral que se caracteriza por la proliferación de elementos gliales y conjuntivo-vasculares.

Cicatrice cérébrale : processus de réparation tissulaire imparfaite consécutive à l'évolution d'une lésion cérébrale et caractérisée par une prolifération neurogliale et conjonctivo-vasculaire.

Cicatriz meningocerebral: cicatriz y adherencias del tejido cerebral y las meninges contiguas.

Cicatrice cérébro-méningée : cicatrice avec adhérences entre le cerveau et les méninges.

Coma: síndrome de inconciencia al cual se agregan en mayor o menor grado alteraciones neurológicas y del sistema autónomo. Se distinguen diversos grados según la presencia y duración de estas alteraciones asociadas.

Coma : état d'inconscience (voir ce terme) associé à des perturbations neurologiques et neurovégétatives plus ou moins importantes. Le degré de gravité dépend de la relativité et de la durée de ces perturbations.

ver: *fractura por compresión.*

Fracture par écrasement : voir *fracture rachidienne par écrasement.*

ver: *parálisis por compresión nerviosa.*

Compression d'un nerf périphérique avec paralysie : voir *paralysie nerveuse par compression.*

14

Concussion, brain-spinal cord: a clinical syndrome characterized by immediate impairment of neural function, such as alteration of consciousness, disturbance of vision, motion, sensation, etc., due to mechanical forces. Although usually transient, more severe grades of concussion may display varying degrees of persistant clinical deficits.

Hirnerschütterung — Rückenmarkserschütterung (im weiteren, im Deutschen nicht gebräuchlichen Sinne): ein klinisches Syndrom — unmittelbar — nach mechanischer Einwirkung auf das Gehirn eintretend, charakterisiert durch sofortige Hirnfunktionsstörungen. Verschiedene Grade der Hirnerschütterung reichen von rascher und vollständiger Rückbildung der Hirnfunktionsstörung (Commotio, Hirnerschütterung im engeren, hier gebräuchlicheren Sinne) bis zu Schweregraden mit irreversiblen Störungen (Contusio cerebri, Hirnprellung).

Confusion: incoherence of thought causing abnormal behavior.

Confusion: ungeordneter Gedankenablauf, der abnormes Verhalten auslöst.

Congestion, brain, spinal cord: increased volume of the intravascular compartment, usually resulting in brain and spinal cord swelling (see also *swelling*, brain).

Hirnstauung (im Deutschen nicht üblich): Vergrößerung des intravasalen Volumenanteiles, was gewöhnlich zur Hirngewebs-Schwellung führt (siehe auch *swelling*, brain).

Consciousness: a state of general wakefulness and awareness of oneself and of responsiveness to environment.

Bewußtseinsklarheit: Zustand uneingeschränkter Wachheit, Wahrnehmung der Umgebung und seiner selbst.

Contrecoup injury of brain: contusion and/or laceration remote from the site of impact.

Gegenstoßherd (Contre-coup), Verletzung des Gehirns: Hirnprellungsherd entgegengesetzt zum Ort der Gewalteinwirkung auf den Schädel.

Conmoción cerebral o medular: sindrome clínico caracterizado por alteración inmediata de la función nerviosa, tal como alteración de la conciencia, de la visión, etc. y debido a fuerzas mecánicas. Aunque generalmente transitoria los grados más severos de conmoción pueden acompañarse de déficits neurológicos persistentes.

Commotion cérébrale, médullaire : syndrome clinique caractérisé par une altération immédiate des fonctions neurologiques, par exemple de la conscience, de la vision, de la motricité, de la sensibilité, consécutif à une atteinte mécanique. Bien que généralement transitoire, une commotion peut cependant entraîner, à des degrés variables, des déficits neurologiques résiduels.

Confusión: incoherencia del pensamiento que causa comportamiento anormal.

Confusion : incohérence de la pensée entraînant un comportement anormal.

Congestión cerebral: aumento de volumen en el compartimiento intra-vascular que produce, habitualmente, hinchazón cerebral (ver *edema cerebral*).

Congestion cérébrale : augmentation de volume du département vasculaire cérébral, engendrant généralement un « gonflement » cérébral (voir aussi *oedème cérébral*).

Conciencia: estado general de vigilia, de percepción del propio ser y de reactividad al ambiente.

Conscience : état de veille et de perception avec réactivité vis-à-vis de l'environnement.

Lesión cerebral por contragolpe: contusión y/o laceración alejada al lugar del impacto.

Traumatisme cérébral par contre-coup : contusion et/ou attrition cérébrale en un autre lieu que l'impact.

Contusion (bruise), brain-spinal cord: a traumatic structural alteration of the neural tissue characterized by extravasation of blood constituents and neural tissue destruction of varying degrees.

Hirnprellung (Hirn-Quetschung), Rückenmarksprellung: traumatische Hirn/Rückenmarksgewebeschädigung, gekennzeichnet durch Austritt von Blutbestandteilen (Extravasaten) und mehr oder weniger starke Gewebszerstörung.

Contusion, nerve: traumatic hemorrhagic extravasation in nerve with or without interruption of axons.

Nervenquetschung: traumatische Blutextravasate in Nerven mit oder ohne Unterbrechung der Axone.

Contusion (bruise), scalp: cutaneous or subcutaneous extravasation of blood without gross disruption of skin.

Prellung (Quetschung) der Kopfschwarte: Blutextravasate in oder unter die Kopfschwarte ohne gröbere Durchtrennung der Haut.

Coup injury of brain, direct: contusion and/or laceration occurring directly beneath the area of impact.

Hirnprellungsherd, direkt: Rindenprellungsherd unmittelbar am Ort der Gewalteinwirkung.

C.T.: see *tomography*, computerized.

C. T.   Computer-Tomographie: siehe *tomography*, computerized.

Delirium, post-traumatic: a state of confusion with agitation, hallucinations, delusions and/or disorientation.

Delir, posttraumatisches: Zustand der Bewußtseinstrübung; Verwirrtheitszustand mit Agitation, Halluzinationen, Wahnvorstellungen und/oder Desorientiertheit.

Dementia, post-traumatic: mental deterioration, may be irreversible or partially or totally reversible.

Demenz, posttraumatische: posttraumatische irreversible hirnorganische Wesensänderung; Persönlichkeitsabbau und intellektuelle Leistungsminderung. Nach H. Wieck streng zu unterscheiden von dem (viel häufigeren) reversiblen Durchgangssyndrom.

Contusión cerebral o medular: alteración estructural traumática del tejido nervioso caracterizada por extravasación sanguínea y destrucción tisular de mayor o menor grado.

Contusion du cerveau, de la moëlle épinière : atteinte organique d'origine traumatique du tissu nerveux caractérisée par une extravasation des éléments sanguins avec destruction plus ou moins importante du parenchyme nerveux.

Contusión de nervio: extravasación hemorrágica traumática en un nervio con o sin interrupción axonal.

Contusion d'un nerf : hémorragie traumatique par extravasation à l'intérieur du nerf avec ou non interruption axonique.

Contusión del cuero cabelludo: extravasación sanguínea cutánea o subcutánea sin grosera alteración de la piel.

Contusion du cuir chevelu : extravasation de sang dans les tissus cutané et sous-cutané du cuir chevelu.

Trauma cerebral directo: contusión y/o laceración que ocurre inmediamente por abajo del área de impacto.

Traumatisme cérébral direct : contusion et/ou attrition cérébrale directement sous-jacentes au siège de l'impact.

C. T.: ver *tomografía computada.*

T. C. : voir *tomographie computérisée.*

Delirio post-traumático: estado de confusión, con agitación, alucinaciones, ilusiones y/o desorientación.

Délire post-traumatique : état confusionnel avec agitation, hallucinations, illusions, désorientation.

Demencia post-traumática: deterioro mental que puede ser definitivo o total o parcialmente reversible.

Démence post-traumatique : détérioration mentale pouvant être définitive, s'améliorer ou régresser complètement.

Discography: X-ray visualization of a disk by injection of an absorbable contrast medium into it.

Diskographie: Röntgen-Darstellung der Bandscheibe durch gezielte Injektion eines resorbierbaren Kontrastmittels.

Discopathy (cervical-dorsal-lumbar-sacral), traumatic: fissuration, laceration and/or fragmentation of the disc and usually of the surrounding ligaments with or without displacement of discal fragments against spinal cord, nerve roots, or ligaments.

Bandscheibenschädigung (zervikal-thorakal-lumbal und sakral); traumatisch: Rißbildung, Zerreißung oder Sequestrierung einer Bandscheibe — gewöhnlich auch des anliegenden Ligaments — mit oder ohne Verlagerung von Bandscheiben-Sequestern in Richtung des Rückenmarkkanals, der Spinalwurzeln.

Disk, herniated: extrusion of discal material from intervertebral space posteriorly, posterolaterally, anteriorly or into the vertebral body. Found in the cervical, dorsal and lumbar spine.

Bandscheiben-Vorfall, Bandscheiben-Hernie: Austritt von (zermürbtem) Bandscheibengewebe aus dem Intervertebralspalt oder in den Wirbelkörper, im Bereich der Hals-, Brust- oder Lendenwirbelsäule.

Disk, protruded: protrusion of discal material from the intervertebral space, posteriorly, posterolaterally or anteriorly. Found in the cervical, dorsal and lumbar spine.

Bandscheiben-Protrusion: Vorwölbung von Bandscheibengewebe aus dem Intervertebralspalt nach dorsal, ventral, dorsolateral; im Bereich der Hals-, (Brust-) und Lendenwirbelsäule vorkommend.

Disk, ruptured: extrusion of discal material through a tear of the anulus, the disk and the ligaments posteriorly, posterolaterally or anteriorly. Found in the cervical, dorsal and lumbar spine.

Bandscheiben-Vorfall, perforierter: Perforation von (zermürbtem) Bandscheiben-Gewebe durch einen Riß im Faserring und Längsband, nach dorsal, dorsolateral oder ventral im Bereich der Hals-, Brust- oder Lendenwirbelsäule.

Discografía: visualización radiológica de un disco intervertebral mediante la inyección, dentro del mismo, de un medio de contraste reabsorbible.

Discopatía (cervical, dorsal, lumbar o sacra) traumática: fisuración, laceración y/o fragmentación del disco, y habitualmente de los ligamentos circundantes, con o sin desplazamiento de fragmentos discales contra la médula, las raices nerviosas o ligamentos vecinos.

Hernia discal: extrusión de material discal del espacio intervertebral hacia atrás, póstero-lateralmente, hacia adelante o dentro de un cuerpo vertebral. Puede encontrarse en la columna cervical, dorsal o lumbar.

Protrusión discal: saliencia discal posterior, pósterolateral o anterior por fuera del espacio intervertebral. Puede encontrarse en la columna cervical, dorsal o lumbar.

Disco roto: extrusion de substancia discal a traves de un desgarro del anillo fibroso hacia atrás, adelante o los lados. Puede ser cervical, dorsal o lumbar.

Discographie : image radiologique d'un disque opacifié par injection d'un produit de contraste.

Discopathie (cervicale, dorsale, lombo-sacrée) traumatique : fissuration et/ou fragmentation d'un disque et généralement des ligaments contígus avec ou sans déplacement du disque vers la moëlle, les racines rachidiennes ou les ligaments.

Hernie discale : migration de tissu discal hors de l'espace intersomatique en direction postérieure, postéro-latérale ou antérieure ou encore dans un corps vertébral. Le siège peut en être cervical, dorsal ou lombaire.

Protrusion discale : protrusion du tissu discal en direction postérieure, postéro-latérale ou antérieure par rapport à l'espace intersomatique. Le siège peut en être cervical, dorsal ou lombaire.

Rupture discale : expulsion du tissu discal à travers une déchirure de l'annulus fibrosus en direction postérieure, postérolatérale ou antérieure. Le siège peut en être cervical, dorsal ou lombaire.

2*

Dislocation, vertebral articular processes: dislocation of one or both articular processes usually with overriding of the inferior articular process of the vertebra above into a position anterior to the superior articular process of the vertebra below. It may be complete (jumped process complex, locked facets).

Luxation der Wirbelsäulengelenkfortsätze: Verlagerung eines oder beider Wirbelgelenkfortsätze; hierbei reitet gewöhnlich der Processus articularis inferior des höheren Wirbels auf dem Prozessus articularis superior des unteren Wirbels. (Es kann sich um eine Luxation oder Subluxation handeln.)

Disorientation, post-traumatic: a state of confusion concerning time and place and one's identity.

Desorientiertheit, posttraumatische: Zustand der Bewußtseinstrübung ohne Orientierung über Person, Ort und Zeit.

Dizziness: an imprecise term describing various subjective symptoms such as faintness, giddiness, lightheadedness or unsteadiness (see also *vertigo*).

Schwindel: ungenauer Ausdruck für verschiedene subjektive Symptome, wie Ohnmacht, Taumeligkeit, Benommenheit, Schwanken (siehe auch *vertigo*).

Drowsiness: state of clouding of consciousness from which the patient may be easily arousable.

Schläfrigkeit: Zustand leicht erweckbarer Bewußtseinstrübung. Dösigkeit, Somnolenz.

Edema, brain, spinal cord: a type of brain or spinal cord swelling characterized by increased volume of the extravascular compartment (see also *swelling*, brain).

Hirnödem, Rückenmarksödem: eine Form der Hirn- oder Rückenmarksschwellung mit Zunahme des extravasalen, extrazellulären Volumens (siehe auch *swelling*, brain).

Dislocación vertebral: desplazamiento traumático, completo o incompleto (subluxación) y en general persistente, de estructuras vertebrales adyacentes.

Dislocación de apófisis articulares vertebrales: dislocación uni o bilateral de las apófisis articulares, generalmente con desplazamiento de la apófisis articular de la vértebra superior hacia adelante en relación al de la vértebra inferior. Puede ser una luxación completa con enganche de las apófisis en posición viciosa.

Desorientación, post-traumática: confusión en relación al tiempo, el espacio y la propia identidad.

Mareo: término inpreciso con el que se describen varios síntomas subjetivos como tener sensación de pérdida inminente del conocimiento, inestabilidad, vacío en la cabeza, dificultad en pensar, o vértigo (ver también *vértigo*).

Sopor o embotamiento: estado de perturbación o depresión de la conciencia del cual el paciente puede ser sacado sin mucha dificultad.

Edema cerebral o medular verdadero: tipo de hinchazón del cerebro o médula caracterizado por aumento volumétrico del espacio extravascular (ver también *swelling, brain-spinal cord*).

Luxation vertébrale : atteinte lésionnelle uni ou bilatérale des articulations vertébrales postérolatérales avec généralement chevauchement de l'apophyse articulaire inférieure de la vertèbre sus-jacente en avant de l'apophyse articulaire supérieure de la vertèbre sous-jacente. La luxation peut être irréductible par manoeuvres externes.

Désorientation temporo-spatiale post-traumatique : état confusionnel concernant le temps et le lieu et la propre identité du sujet.

Sensations vertigineuses : terme imprécis recouvrant un ensemble de syndromes subjectifs tels que tendance lypothymique, malaises, « tête vide », instabilité (voir aussi *vertiges*).

Somnolence, obnubilation : diminution du niveau de conscience qui cesse aisément par réveil du sujet.

Oedème cérébral, médullaire : « gonflement » cérébral ou médullaire caractérisé par une augmentation de volume du département extra-vasculaire.

Emphysema, subgaleal: see *pneumocele*, extracranial.

Empyema: collection of pus in preformed spaces, actual or potential, such as subdural, extradural (see also abscess).

Encephalitis: see *cerebritis*.

Emphysem, subgaleales: siehe *pneumocele*, extracranial.

Empyem: Eiteransammlung in vorgebildeten — bestehenden oder möglichen — Gewebsräumen, wie z. B. subdural, epidural (siehe auch *abscess*).

Enzephalitis: siehe *cerebritis*.

Encephalopathy, traumatic chronic (traumatic chronic brain syndrome): chronic disturbance of structure and/or function of nerve cells, glia, or intracranial vessels resulting from injury and characterized by mental and some motor disorders, sometimes progressive.

Entrapment: the compression of nerves and/or vessels in their course through deformed or hypertrophied musculoskeletal structures.

Epidural (extradural) hemorrhage, craniocerebral-spinal: see *hematoma*, epidural (extradural); in hematoma, craniocerebral-spinal.

Epilepsy, post-traumatic: epilepsy after a brain injury and caused by it. The onset can be early (for instance during the first month, late and sometimes very late (see also *seizures*, post-traumatic).

Enzephalopathie, traumatische, chronische (posttraumatisches hirnorganisches Syndrom): posttraumatische Störung von Aufbau und/oder Funktion von Nervenzellen, Glia oder intrakraniellen Gefäßen, mit psychischen und neurologischen Störungen.

Einschnürung: Kompression von Nerven und/oder Gefäßen während ihres Verlaufes durch deformierte oder verdickte muskuläre — bindegewebige — knöcherne Strukturen.

Epidurales (extradurales) Hämatom, intrakraniell-intraspinal: siehe *hematoma*, epidural.

Epilepsie, posttraumatische: hirnorganische Anfälle nach Hirntraumen. Der Beginn kann früh (z. B. während des ersten Monates), spät oder manchmal sehr spät liegen (siehe auch *seizures*, post-traumatic).

Enfisema subgaleal: ver *pneumo-cele extracraneal.*

Empiema: colección de pus en un espacio preformado, actual o en potencia, como el subdural o el extradural (ver también *absceso*).

Encefalitis: ver *cerebritis.*

Encefalopatía, crónica traumática (síndrome cerebral crónico post-traumático): alteración estructur-al y/o funcional crónica de las neuronas, la glia y/o los vasos cerebrales de origen traumático que se caracteriza por trastornos mentales, y a veces motores, que pueden ser progresivos.

Atrapamiento: compresión de ner-vios y/o vasos en su trayecto a través de estructural músculo-esqueléticas deformadas o hiper-trofiadas.

Hemorragia epidural (extradural) craniocerebral-espinal: ver *he-matoma epidural o extradural* en: *Hematoma craniocerebral-espinal.*

Epilepsia post-traumática: epilep-sia consecutiva a una lesión cere-bral y causada por la misma. El comienzo puede ser precoz (por ej. en el primer mes), tardío o muy tardío (ver también *con-vulsiones o ataques post-trau-máticos*).

Emphysème du cuir chevelu : voir *pneumocèle extracranien.*

Empyème : collection de pus dans un espace préformé, présent ou virtuel, tel que l'espace sous-dural, l'espace extra-dural (voir aussi *abcès*).

Encéphalite : état inflammatoire du cerveau pouvant évoluer ou non vers un état suppuratif.

Encéphalopathie chronique, post-traumatique : perturbation chro-nique de la structure et/ou de la fonction des cellules nerveuses, gliales ou des vaisseaux intra-crâniens due à un traumatisme et caractérisée par des troubles mentaux et moteurs parfois pro-gressifs.

Incarcération : compression de nerfs et/ou de vaisseaux durant leur trajet au travers des struc-tures ostéomusculaires déformées ou hypertrophiées.

Hématome extra-dural crânien, spinal : voir dans la rubrique : *hématome intracranien, intra-rachidien.*

Epilepsie post-traumatique : épi-lepsie apparaissant après un traumatisme cérébral et sous sa dépendance. Le début peut en être précoce (par exemple pen-dant le 1er mois), tardif ou ul-tra-tardif (voir aussi *crises épi-leptiques post-traumatiques*).

Fibrositis, cervical-dorsal-lumbar: inflamación del tejido fibrosa en la musculatura espinal (ver también *síndrome cervical post-traumático*).

Fibrose, cervicale, dorsale, lombaire : (terme non usité) inflammation du tissu fibreux de la musculature spinale (fibrose inflammatoire).

Fistula carotido-cavernosa post-traumática: comunicación arteriovenosa por ruptura de la porción intracavernosa de la carótida interna o de sus pequeñas ramas.

Fistule carotido-caverneuse post-traumatique : communication artério-veineuse résultant de la rupture du segment intra-caverneux de la carotide.

Fractura de la base del cráneo.

Fracture de la base du crâne : fracture intéressant la base du crâne.

Fractura cerrada de cráneo: verlo en *craniocerebral injury*.

Fracture fermée du crâne : voir ce terme dans la rubrique : *traumatismes cranio-cérébraux*.

Fractura cerrada (simple) de columna: fractura sin lesión de las partes blandas superficiales.

Fracture fermée du rachis : fracture rachidienne sans lésions des tissus mous.

Fractura conminuta de cráneo o columna: fractura con fragmentación ósea.

Fracture comminutive du crâne, du rachis : fracture multi-fragmentaire.

Fractura de columna por compresión: aplastamiento del cuerpo vertebral, por lo común mayor en su parte anterior.

Fracture rachidienne par écrasement : 1. le corps de la vertèbre est généralement plus écrasé en avant qu'en arrière. 2. Tassement du corps vertébral généralement plus important en avant d'où un aspect trapézoïdal. 3. Ecrasement presque complet des éléments vertébraux et intervertébraux.

Fracture, depressed, skull: fracture with inward displacement of the calvarium. The so-called "dishpan", "derby hat", and "ping pong" fractures consist of smooth cranial concavity in infants and may or may not be associated with fracture.

Impressionsfraktur des Schädels: Einwärtsverlagerung von Knochenfragmenten. Die sogenannte „Tischtennisball"-Fraktur entsteht am elastischen Schädelknochen der Kinder mit oder ohne Kontinuitätstrennung.

Fracture, depressed, spine: fracture with displacement of bone toward spinal canal.

Wirbel-Kompressions-Fraktur mit Verlagerung von Knochenfragmenten in den Wirbelkanal.

Fracture, diastatic, skull: 1. separation of cranial bones at a suture; 2. fracture with marked separation of bone fragments.

Schädelkalotten-Berstungsfraktur: durch 1. Nahtsprengung, 2. „klaffende" Kalotten-Stückfraktur.

Fracture, "dishpan", "Derby hat", and "ping pong": see *fracture, depressed skull.*

Tischtennisball-/Ping-Pong-Ball-Fraktur: siehe *fracture,* depressed skull (die anderen Bezeichnungen sind im Deutschen nicht gebräuchlich).

Fracture, dislocation, spine: a break with displacement of broken elements. Tear of joint elements permits displacement.

Wirbel-Luxationsfraktur: Verlagerung von Frakturelementen durch das gleichzeitige Zerreißen von Gelenkanteilen ermöglicht.

Fracture, expressed (exploded), skull: fracture with outward displacement of the cranium.

Expressions-Fraktur: mit Auswärtsverlagerung von Fragmenten.

Fractura deprimida de cráneo: fractura con desplazamiento hacia adentro de parte del calvario. La fractura „en palangana" o de „ping-pong" en primera infancia consiste en una concavidad regular del cráneo que puede asociarse o nó con fractura.

Embarrure : fracture avec déplacement intra-crânien des fragments. Les enfoncements dits en « balle de ping-pong » correspondent à une déformation en cupule du crâne encore mou de l'enfant et peuvent ou non comporter véritablement une fracture.

Fractura deprimida de columna: fractura con desplazamiento de hueso hacia el conducto espinal.

Fracture rachidienne avec atteinte du mur postérieur : fracture avec déplacement vers le canal spinal de la paroi vertébrale postérieure.

Fractura craneana con diástasis: la separación ósea puede hacerse a nivel de una sutura (falsa fractura) o de los fragmentos óseos.

Fracture crânienne avec déhiscence : 1. Des sutures : fracture avec séparation et parfois écartement des os du crâne au niveau des sutures. 2. Des fragments osseux.

Fracture, „dishpan", „derby hat", „ping pong": ver *fractura deprimida de cráneo.*

Fracture en cupule, en balle de « ping-pong » : voir *embarrure.*

Fractura-dislocación de columna: la ruptura ligamentosa permite el desplazamiento de los fragmentos óseos.

Fracture-luxation du rachis : fracture du rachis avec déplacement de l'axe rachidien. L'atteinte ligamentaire permet ces déplacements.

Fractura exprimida del cráneo: fractura con desplazamiento hacia afuera de los fragmentos óseos.

Fracture extériorisée : fracture avec déplacement vers l'extérieur des fragments osseux (terme non usité).

28

Fracture, fulcrum (chance): horizontal fracture through vertebra, vertebral body and other elements of the vertebra horizontally broken and torn. Usually seen in auto accidents and lap belt injury.

Dreh-, Torsions-Wirbelbruch: horizontaler Bruch und Drehung des Wirbels und seiner Einzel-Elemente, gewöhnlich bei Auto-Unfällen und Beckengurt-Verletzungen.

Fracture, hangman's: fracture of axis and third cervical vertebra with break of neural arch of the axis and detachment of the body of the axis from the third cervical vertebra. The neural arch of the axis continues to be attached to the third cervical while the body of the axis is attached to the atlas. One or both pedicles of third cervical vertebra may be fractured.

Henker-Fraktur: Bruch des 2. und 3. Halswirbels mit Bruch des Axis-Bogens, welcher am 3. Wirbel hängen bleibt, und Lösung des mit dem Atlas verbundenen Axis-Körpers vom 3. Wirbel. Ein oder beide Gelenkfortsätze des 3. Wirbels können dabei brechen.

Fracture, linear, skull-spine: a fracture resembling a line.

Linear-Fraktur von Schädel-Wirbelsäule: linienförmiger Bruch.

Fracture, open skull (compound): see *skull fracture,* open in *craniocerebral injury.*

Schädelbruch, offener (komplizierter): siehe *skull fracture,* open in *craniocerebral injury.*

Fracture, open spine (compound): a fracture with laceration of overlying soft tissues.

Wirbelbruch, offener (komplizierter): Wirbelbruch mit Zerreißung der darüberliegenden Weichteile.

Fracture, progressive: 1. enlarging fracture due to the pulsatile force of cerebro-spinal fluid in spurious cranial meningocele; 2. widening fracture due to loss of periosteal lining.

Wachsende Schädelfraktur: 1. infolge der Liquorpulsation bei Schädelfraktur mit Dura-Hirn-Verletzung und Ventrikel-Eröffnung; 2. klaffende Fraktur infolge Verlust des anliegenden Periostes.

Fractura en fulcro: fractura transversal de una vértebra. El cuerpo y otros segmentos vertebrales pueden romperse horizontalmente con separación de los fragmentos, generalmente en accidente de auto con cinturón de seguridad.

Fracture vertébrale horizontale : fracture horizontale du corps vertébral. Les autres éléments vertébraux peuvent être fracturés ou déchirés horizontalement. Cette fracture survient généralement lors des accidents de voiture avec port de la ceinture de sécurité.

Fractura de ahorcado: fractura del arco neural del axis y separación del cuerpo del axis de la 3ª vértebra. El arco posterior del axis continúa adherido a la 3ª vértebra y el cuerpo del mismo queda adherido al atlas. Uno o ambos pedículos de la 3ª vértebra pueden fracturarse.

Fracture du pendu : fracture de l'axis et de la 3ème vertèbre cervicale avec rupture de l'arc postérieur de l'axis et des attaches du corps de l'axis avec la 3ème vertèbre cervicale. L'arc postérieur conserve ses attaches avec la 3ème vertèbre cervicale et le corps de l'axis les siennes avec l'atlas. Les deux pédicules de la 3ème vertèbre, ou un seul, sont fracturés.

Fractura linear (de cráneo o vértebra).

Fracture linéaire du crâne, du rachis : fracture en ligne.

Fractura expuesta de cráneo: ver en *trauma encefalocraneano.*

Fracture ouverte du crâne : voir ce terme dans la rubrique *traumatismes cranio-cérébraux.*

Fractura expuesta de columna: fractura con laceración de tejidos superficiales.

Fracture rachidienne ouverte : fracture avec plaie des tissus mous de recouvrement.

Fractura progresiva: 1. fractura que se agranda a causa de la fuerza pulsátil del líquido cefalo-raquídeo en un falso meningocele craneano traumático; 2. fractura que se ensancha por pérdida de su revestimiento perióstico.

Fracture évolutive : (terme non usité) 1. Fracture s'élargissant du fait de la force pulsatile du l. c. r. d'un faux méningocèle. 2. Trait de fracture s'élargissant du fait de la perte de revêtement périosté.

Fracture, spine: break of vertebra and/or its elements (body, pedicles, transverse processes, lamina and spinous process) resulting from trauma.

Wirbelbruch: traumatischer Bruch eines Wirbels und/oder seiner Bestandteile (Körper-, Bögen-, Quer-, Gelenk- und Dornfortsätze).

Fracture, stellate, skull: multiple linear fractures radiating from the area of impact.

Sternfraktur des Schädeldaches: vom Ort der Gewalteinwirkung sternförmig auslaufende Fraktur-Linien.

Fracture "tear drop": sprain fracture of the vertebral body with small anterior-inferior portion of bone adjacent to the ligaments pulled off.

„Tränen-Tropfen-Fraktur" des **Wirbels:** Abriß eines schmalen Fragmentes der vorderen unteren Wirbelkörperkante, haftend am vorderen Längsband.

Fungus, cerebri: ulcerated cerebral hernia.

Hirnprolaps: bruchartige Ausstülpung (Vorfall) des Hirns und seiner Häute durch einen Knochendefekt.

Graft, bone, skull-spine: usually autologous bone used to correct a defect or to fuse bony structures.

Knochentransplantat, Schädel-, Wirbel-: gewöhnlich autologes Knochenstück zur Defektdeckung oder zur Vereinigung von Knochen-Strukturen.

Graft, nerve: usually autologous nerve used to repair a gap caused by extensive injury.

Nerventransplantat: gewöhnlich autologes Nervenstück zur Überbrückung eines Defektes bei ausgedehnter Verletzung.

Graft, skin: usually autologous skin to cover a defect of the skin layer. Heterologous grafts may be used in certain skin lesions, e.g., burns.

Hauttransplantat: gewöhnlich autologes Hautstück zur Deckung eines Hautdefektes. Heterologe Hauttransplantate können z. B. bei Hautverbrennungen benutzt werden.

Fractura de columna: fractura de una o más vértebras (o de sus elementos) de origen traumático.

Fracture du rachis : fracture de la vertèbre ou de ses éléments (corps, pédicules, apophyses transverses, lames et apophyses articulaires) consécutive à un traumatisme.

Fractura estrellada de cráneo: múltiples fracturas lineares radiantes desde el area de impacto.

Fracture du crâne en étoile : fracture avec de multiples traits en rayons à partir du point d'impact.

Fractura "en gota": fractura por arrancamiento de un pequeño trozo ántero-inferior del cuerpo vertebral.

Fracture en larme : arrachement par les ligaments d'un petit fragment osseux au niveau du coin antéro-inférieur d'un corps vertébral.

Fungus cerebral: hernia cerebral ulcerada.

Fungus cérébral : hernie cérébrale ulcérée.

Injerto oseo de cráneo o columna: generalmente de hueso autólogo, para corregir un defecto o unir estructuras óseas.

Greffe osseuse crânienne, rachidienne : plastie d'une perte de substance ou fusion de structures osseuses par un fragment d'os, généralement prélevé sur l'individu lui-même (autogène).

Injerto de nervio: generalmente de nervio autólogo para reparar un defecto causado por lesión extensa.

Greffe nerveuse : utilisation d'un fragment de nerf, généralement prélevé sur l'individu lui-même (autogène), pour réparer une perte de substance traumatique d'un nerf.

Injerto cutáneo: generalmente de piel autóloga para cubrir un defecto de los tegumentos. Injertos heterólogos pueden usarse en ciertas lesiones cutáneas, por ej. en quemaduras.

Greffe cutanée : utilisation d'un greffon cutané généralement prélevé sur l'individu lui-même (autogène) pour recouvrir une perte de substance cutanée. Des fragments de peau hétérogène peuvent être utilisés dans certaines lésions cutanées en particulier consécutives à des brûlures.

Halter traction: see *traction*, halter.

Headache, tension: see *syndrome*, neck, post-traumatic.

Hematoma, craniocerebral-spinal: local collection of blood, may be *epidural* (*extradural*) *subdural*, in the brain (*intracerebral*), in the spinal cord (*hematomyelia*). It may be acute (one day) subacute (two or ten days), or chronic (more than eleven days).

Hematomyelia: hemorrhage in the spinal cord (see also *hematoma*).

Hematorrhachis (or hemorrhachis): hemorrhage into the spinal canal.

Hemorrhage, subarachnoid, intracranial-spinal, traumatic: extravasation of blood into the subarachnoid space. The blood spreads throughout the space along cerebrospinal fluid pathways; but may remain as localized accumulations in certain areas.

Herniated disk: see *disk*, herniated.

Herniation, cingulate: displacement of cingulate gyrus beneath the falx.

Herniation, foraminal (tonsillar): displacement of cerebellar tonsils through the foramen magnum.

Halter-Extension: siehe *traction*, halter.

Kopfschmerz durch reflektorische Muskelverspannung: siehe *syndrome*, neck, post-traumatic.

Hämatom, Blutung, intrakraniell-spinal: örtliche Blutansammlung, die epidural (extradural), subdural, intra-zerebral bzw. intramedullär (Hämatomyelie) liegen kann. Verlauf akut (1 Tag), subakut (2—10 Tage) oder chronisch (mehr als 10 Tage).

Hämatomyelie: intramedulläre Blutung (siehe auch *hematoma*).

Hämatorrhachis: intraspinale Blutung.

Subarachnoidalblutung, traumatische, des Gehirns oder des Rückenmarks: Blutung in den Subarachnoidalraum, breitet sich entlang den Liquorwegen aus, aber kann auch auf bestimmte Gebiete lokal raumfordernd begrenzt bleiben.

Bandscheibenvorfall: siehe *disk*, herniated.

Gyrus-Cinguli-Prolaps: Verlagerung des Gyrus cinguli unter die Falx cerebri auf Grund der Massenverschiebung.

Kleinhirntonsillen-Prolaps (Druckkonus) in das Foramen occipitale magnum. Hinterhauptsloch-Einklemmung.

Tracción confronda o cabestrillo: ver *tracción* cervical.

Traction par fronde : voir *fronde.*

Cefalea por tension: ver *síndrome cervical post-traumático.*

Céphalées postérieures : voir *syndrome cervical post-traumatique.*

Hematoma intracraneano o espinal: colección sanguínea localizada. Puede ser extradural (epidural), subdural, intracerebral o intramedular (hematomielia). Puede ser agudo (un día), subagudo (2 a 10 días) o crónico (11 o más días).

Hématome intra-crânien, intra-rachidien : collection de sang dont le siège peut être extra-dural (épidural), sous-dural, in-tra-cérébral, dans la moelle épinière (hématomyélie). L'hématome peut être aigu (le 1er jour), sub-aigu (du 2ème au 10ème jour) ou chronique (après le 11ème jour).

Hematomielia: hemorragia intramedular. Ver también *hematoma.*

Hématomyélie : hémorragie dans la moelle épinière (voir aussi *hématome*).

Hematorraquis: hemorragia en el conducto raquídeo.

Hématorrachis (ou hémorrachis) : hémorragie à l'intérieur du canal rachidien.

Hemorragia subaracnoidea, intra-traneana-espinal, traumática: extravasación de sangre en los espacios subaracnoideos. La sangre se difunde en el líquido cefalorraquídeo pero puede quedar tambien localizada en ciertas áreas.

Hémorragie sous-arachnoïdienne, intra-crânienne, rachidienne, post-traumatique : épanchement de sang dans les espaces sous-arachnoïdiens. Le sang se répand dans ces espaces en suivant le cheminement du l. c. r., mais peut rester aussi localisé en certains points.

Hernia discal: ver *disco*, hernia.

Hernie discale : voir ce terme.

Hernia del cingulum o hernia subfalcial: desplazamiento del girus cinguli bajo la hoz del cerebro.

Hernie ou engagement cingulaire (sous la faux) : déplacement latéral du gyrus cingulaire sous la faux.

Hernia foraminal o amigdalina: desplazamiento de las amígdalas cerebelosas a través del foramen magnum.

Hernie ou engagement amygdalien : déplacement d'une ou des amygdales cérébelleuses vers le bas au travers du trou occipital.

34

Herniation, transtentorial, caudal:
displacement of medial temporal structures into incisura with or without lateral and rostrocaudal brain stem shift.

Temporaler oder tentorieller Druckkonus: Tentoriumschlitz-Einklemmung, Uncus-Prolaps. Verlagerung medio-temporaler Strukturen in die Incisura tentorii mit oder ohne lateraler oder rostro-caudaler Hirnstamm-Verlagerung.

Herniation, transtentorial, rostral:
displacement of anterior cerebellar structures into incisura, with or without lateral caudorostral brain stem shift.

Cerebellärer Druckkonus nach oben: cerebelläre Tentoriumschlitz-Einklemmung. Verlagerung oberer Kleinhirn-Anteile nach rostral in die Incisura tentorii mit oder ohne lateraler oder caudo-rostraler Hirnstammverlagerung.

Hydrocephalus, post-meningitic:
ventricular dilation following meningitis and secondary to obstruction of cerebrospinal fluid pathways.

Hydrocephalus, postmeningitischer: Hirnkammer-Erweiterung nach Meningitis und infolge Verlegung der liquorableitenden Wege.

Hydrocephalus, post-traumatic:
ventricular dilation caused by brain injury, brain atrophy, and impaired cerebrospinal fluid circulation and/or pressure.

Hydrocephalus, posttraumatischer: Hirnkammererweiterung nach Hirntrauma infolge Hirnatrophie und Störungen von Liquor-Zirkulation und/oder Druck.

Hydrocephalus, "ex-vacuo": inappropriate term-should not be used. Enlargement of the ventricle into an area of brain atrophy or traumatic skull defect and brain injury.

Hydrocephalus „ex vacuo": unrichtiger, daher nicht zu benutzender Ausdruck.

Hernia transtentorial descendente (caudal): desplazamiento de las estructuras temporales medias a través del borde libre de la tienda del cerebelo con o sin desplazamiento contralateral y caudal del tronco cerebral.

Hernie ou engagement temporal : déplacement des structures temporales internes à travers l'incisure tentorielle avec ou sans refoulement en dedans et vers le bas du tronc cérébral.

Hernia transtentorial ascendente (rostral): desplazamiento de las estructuras cerebelosas superiores a través de la tienda del cerebelo con o sin desplazamiento lateral y rostral del tronco cerebral.

Hernie cérébelleuse supérieure : déplacement de la partie antéro-supérieure des structures cérébelleuses à travers l'incisure tentorielle avec ou sans refoulement latéral et vers le haut du tronc cérébral.

Hidrocefalia post-meningitis: dilatación ventricular consecutiva a una meningitis por bloqueo de las vías del líquido céfalo-raquídeo.

Hydrocéphalie post-méningitique : dilatation ventriculaire consécutive à une méningite et due à une obstruction des voies de cheminement du l. c. r.

Hidrocefalia post-traumática: dilatación ventricular causada por trauma cerebral y generalmente debida a alteraciones de la circulación del líquido céfalo-raquídeo y/o de la presión intra-craneana.

Hydrocéphalie post-traumatique : dilatation ventriculaire consécutive à un traumatisme cérébral, une atrophie cérébrale, une perturbation de la circulation ou de la pression du l. c. r.

Hidrocefalia ex-vacuo: término inapropiado que no debe usarse.

Hydrocéphalie a vacuo : terme impropre, à ne pas utiliser.

3*

Hydroma, hygroma, subdural, intracranial, traumatic: accumulation in the subdural space of cerebrospinal fluid, frequently with modified composition. It may be acute or chronic.

Hydrom, Hygrom, subdurales, traumatisches: Subdurale Ansammlung von Liquor, oft veränderter Zusammensetzung, akut oder chronisch.

Hyperextension-hyperflexion injury, cervical: see *injury*, hyperextension-hyperflexion, cervical.

Zervikales Hyperextensions-Hyperflexions-Trauma: siehe *injury*, hyperextension-hyperflexion, cervical.

Injury, head: see *craniocerebral* injury.

Schädel-Hirntrauma: siehe *craniocerebral* injury.

Injury, hyperextension-hyperflexion, cervical: a term to indicate violence to the body causing the unsupported head to hyperextend and/or hyperflex the neck rapidly without direct impact. It should not be used to imply any specific resultant pathological condition or syndrome.

Zervikales Hyperextensions-Hyperflexions-Trauma: Bezeichnung für eine Gewalteinwirkung auf den Körper, bei welcher der unfixierte Kopf eine schnelle Überstreckung und/oder Überbeugung des Halses, ohne direkte Einwirkung auf diesen, ausführen läßt. Der Ausdruck sollte nicht benutzt werden, um irgendeine hieraus resultierende spezifische pathologische Veränderung oder ein Syndrom zu bezeichnen.

Injury "whiplash": a popular term for hyperextension-hyperflexion injuries. The term should not be used to imply any specific resultant pathological condition or syndrome.

Peitschenhieb-Verletzung der Halswirbelsäule: populärer Ausdruck für Hyperextensions-Hyperflexions-Traumen. Siehe dort.

Hidroma, higroma, subdural, intracraneano, traumático: acumulación en el espacio subdural de L. C. R. cuya composición está frecuentemente alterada. Puede ser agudo o crónico.

ver: *traumatismo cervical por hiperextensión-hiperflexión.*

Trauma cefálico: ver *trauma encéfalo-craneano.*

Traumatismo cervical por hiperextensión-hiperflexión: términos que indican violencia corporal que provoca la hiperextensión y/o la hiperflexión de la cabeza y cuello sin apoyo. Estos términos no deben usarse como significando un sindrome específico o una patología determinada.

Traumatismo cervical „en latigazo": término popular para los traumas en hiperextensión-hiperflexión.

Hydrome (hygrome) sous-dural, intra-crânien post-traumatique: accumulation de l. c. r. dans l'espace sous-dural avec généralement modification des constantes biologiques de ce l. c. r. L'hydrome peut être aigu ou chronique.

Traumatisme cervical par hyperextension, par hyperflexion: voir ce terme.

Traumatisme crânien: voir ce terme dans la rubrique: *traumatismes cranio-cérébraux.*

Traumatisme cervical par hyperextension, par hyperflexion: un déplacement rapide du corps est susceptible d'entraîner, du fait de l'absence de fixité de l'extrémité céphalique, une brutale hyperextension ou hyperflexion du cou sans impact direct. Ce terme ne doit pas être utilisé pour décrire les résultats pathologiques de ce traumatisme ou un syndrome.

Coup de fouet cervical, coup de fléau cervical: terme couramment utilisé pour désigner les traumatismes cervicaux par hyperextension et/ou hyperflexion. Le terme « coup du lapin » est souvent utilisé, mais en principe devrait être réservé aux cas où un impact direct sur le rachis cervical est en cause. Ces termes ne doivent pas être utilisés pour décrire les résultats pathologiques du traumatisme ou un syndrome.

Intracerebral hematoma: see *hematoma*, intracerebral, in *hematoma* craniocerebral.

Interval, free, lucid: transient period of relative well being followed by severe neurological deteriotion. It may be preceded by initial unconsciousness following the head injury.

Jumped process complex: see dislocation, vertebral articular processes.

Laceration, brain-spinal cord: lesion characterized by gross tearing of neural tissue and its vasculature (see also *wound*).

Leptomeningeal cyst, post-traumatic (meningocele): a subcutaneous persistent cystic accumulation of cerebro-spinal fluid with progressive loss of bone and dura, occuring at the site of a previous fracture with dura and brain lesion (see also *fracture*, progressive).

Leptomeningeal fibrosis: see *arachnoiditis*, adhesive.

Leptomeningitis: see *meningitis*, traumatic.

List: a popular terme to indicate inclination of the spine laterally, anteriorly and/or posteriorly due to muscular spasm.

Intrazerebrales Hämatom: siehe *hematoma*, intracerebral, in *hematoma* craniocerebral.

Intervall, freies: symptomfreier Zeitraum zwischen Trauma und späterem Einsetzen einer Hämatom-Symptomatologie.

Subluxationssyndrom: siehe dislocation, vertebral articular processes.

Lazeration des Gehirns, des Rückenmarks: grobe Zerreißung von Hirn- und Rückenmarksgewebe und -gefäßen (siehe auch *wound*).

Leptomeningeale Zyste, falsche Meningozele, posttraumatische: im Deutschen nicht mehr gebräuchliche Bezeichnung für die wachsende Schädelfraktur (siehe auch *fracture*, progressive).

Leptomeningeale Fibrose (ungebräuchlich): siehe *arachnoiditis*, adhesive.

Leptomeningitis: siehe *meningitis*, traumatic.

Schlagseite: im Deutschen ungebräuchliche Bezeichnung für seitliche Vorwärts- oder Rückwärts-Schiefhaltung der Wirbelsäule bei Muskelspasmus. Hier vergleichbar: Hexenschuß.

ver: *hematoma* intracerebral en *hematoma* craneocerebral.

Hématome intracérébral : voir ce terme dans la rubrique: *Hematome intracrânien.*

Intervalo lúcido o libre: período transitorio de relativo bienestar seguido por seria agravación neurológica. Puede ser precedido por inconciencia inicial.

Intervalle libre : état transitoire relativement satisfaisant, suivi d'une importante aggravation. Il peut être précédé par une perte de connaissance initiale.

ver: *dislocación de facetas articulares vertebrales.*

Luxation vertébrale : voir ce terme.

Laceración de cerebro o médula: lesión caracterizada por desgarramiento grosero del tejido nervioso y sus vasos (ver también *wound*).

Plaie, attrition, cérébrale, médullaire : Lésion caractérisée par une destruction directe du parenchyme nerveux et des vaisseaux.

Quiste leptomeníngeo (meningocele) post-traumático: acumulación subcutánea, quística y persistente, de L. C. R. con pérdida progresiva de hueso y dura a nivel de una antigua fractura con lesión de dura y cerebro (ver también *fractura* progresiva).

Faux méningocèle post-traumatique : voir ce terme.

Fibrosis leptomeníngea: ver *aracnoiditis* adhesiva.

Arachnoïdite adhésive : voir ce terme.

Leptomeningitis: ver *meningitis* traumática.

Leptoméningite : voir *méningite post-traumatique.*

List: término popular sin traducción médica apropiada que indica una inclinación de la columna vertebral, en cualquier dirección, por espasmo muscular.

De guingois : terme populaire pour désigner une inclinaison latérale antérieure et/ou postérieure de la colonne rachidienne consécutive à une contracture musculaire.

Locked facets: dislocation of facet joints not reduced by traction; see *dislocation*, vertebral articular process.

Luxation: dislocation. Term generally not used.

Meningitis (leptomeningitis), traumatic: inflammation of the piarachnoid, caused by germ propagation through a craniocerebral open brain injury. It may be early or late.

Meningitis, serous: see *hydroma*.

Meningocele, spurious (traumatic), head: see *leptomeningeal cyst*.

Meningocele, spurious (traumatic) spinal: extraspinal cerebrospinal fluid accumulation due to traumatic meningeal tear.

Myelitis, spinal cord: inflammation of spinal cord.

Myelitis, traumatic: bruise, hemorrhage, or section of spinal cord with varying degrees of functional disturbance.

Locked facets: Luxation der kleinen Wirbelgelenke, die durch Extension nicht beseitigt werden kann (siehe *dislocation*, vertebral articular process).

Luxation: im Deutschen gebräuchlich, im Englischen ungebräuchliche Bezeichnung (siehe *dislocation*, locked facets).

Meningitis (Leptomeningitis), posttraumatische: Entzündung der weichen Hirnhäute infolge Eindringens von Erregern durch eine offene Hirnverletzung. Kann früh oder spät auftreten.

Meningitis, seröse: siehe *hydroma*.

Falsche Meningozele, wachsende Schädelfraktur: siehe *fracture*, progressive, *leptomeningeal cyst*.

Meningozele, falsche (traumatische), spinale: Liquoransammlung außerhalb des Spinalkanals infolge Zerreißung der Hirnhäute.

Myelitis: Rückenmarksentzündung.

Myelitis, traumatische: im Deutschen ungebräuchliche Bezeichnung für Quetschung oder Blutung des Rückenmarks.

Faceta articular trabada: ver *dislocación de procesos articulares vertebrales.*

Luxation rachidienne fixée : luxation irréductible par traction.

Luxación: sinónimo de dislocación.

Luxation : voir *luxation vertébrale.*

Meningitis (leptomeningitis) traumática: inflamación pioaracnoidea causada por propagación de gérmenes a través de una herida craneocerebral abierta. Puede ser precoz o tardía.

Méningite (leptoméningite) post-traumatique : inflammation de la pie-arachnoïde, due à des germes se propageant à travers la brèche d'un traumatisme craniocérébral ouvert. La méningite peut être précoce ou tardive.

Meningitis serosa: ver *hidroma.*

Méningite séreuse : voir *hydrome.*

Meningocele espurio (traumático) cefálico: ver *quiste leptomeníngeo.*

Faux méningocèle post-traumatique : accumulation persistante de l. c. r. dans les tissus sous-cutanés avec érosion progressive du crâne et de la dure-mère, se produisant au niveau d'une fracture pré-existante avec brèche durale et osseuse.

Meningocele espurio (traumático) raquídeo: acumulación extradural de L. C. R. por desgarramiento meníngeo traumático.

Faux méningocèle rachidien : accumulation de l. c. r. en dehors du fourreau dural consécutive à une plaie méningée.

Myélite : état inflammatoire de la moelle épinière.

Mielitis traumática: contusión, hemorragia o sección medular con grados variables de alteración funcional.

Lésion médullaire traumatique : écrasement, hémorragie, section de la moëlle épinière avec degrés variés de perturbations fonctionnelles.

Myelopathy, traumatic: chronic and sometimes changing post-traumatic spinal cord disturbance.

Myelopathie, traumatisch: chronische, manchmal wechselnde posttraumatische Rückenmarksschädigung.

Neck syndrome, post-traumatic: see *syndrome*, neck, post-traumatic.

Zervikalsyndrom, posttraumatisches: siehe *syndrome*, neck, post-traumatic.

Nerve anastomosis: see *anastomosis*, nerve.

Nervennaht: siehe *neurorrhaphie*.

Nerve entrapment: see *entrapment*.

Nerveneinschnürung: siehe *entrapment*.

Nerve graft: see *graft*, nerve.

Nerventransplantat: siehe *graft*, nerve.

Nerve overlap: partial compensation of nerve function from an adjoining area of nerve distribution in case of nerve section or compression. May be sensory and motor.

Nerven-Überlappung: partielle Kompensation einer sensiblen oder motorischen Nervenfunktion durch das Ausbreitungsgebiet eines dem verletzten Nerv benachbarten Nerven.

Nerve transplant: see *graft*, nerve.

Nerventransplantat: siehe *graft*, nerve.

Neuralgia, occipital (suboccipital), traumatic: see *syndrome*, neck, post-traumatic.

Okzipitalis-Neuralgie (Subokzipitalis-), traumatische: siehe *syndrome*, neck, post-traumatic.

Neuralgia, sciatic: pain in distribution of sciatic nerve (lower back, one or both lower limbs). May be traumatic.

Ischialgie: Schmerzen im Ausbreitungsgebiet der unteren Lumbalwurzeln, evtl. traumatisch.

Neuralgia, trigeminal: syndrome of reoccuring paroxysmal pain in the distribution of the trigeminal nerve or one or more of its branches. Rarely traumatic.

Trigeminusneuralgie: rezidivierende Schmerzanfälle im Gebiet eines oder mehrerer Trigeminus-Äste. Selten traumatisch.

Mielopatia traumática: alteración medular crónica, y a veces cambiante, de origen traumático.

ver: *síndrome* cervical post-traumático.

ver: *anastomosis* de nervio.

ver: *atrapamiento* nervioso.

ver: *injerto* nervioso.

Superposición territorial nerviosa: compensación parcial de la función de un nervio por otro vecino en caso de compresión o sección. Puede ser sensitiva o motora.

Transplante de nervio: ver *injerto* de nervio.

Neuralgia, occipital (suboccipital), traumatica: ver *síndrome* cervical post-traumático.

Neuralgia ciática: dolor en el territorio del nervio ciático (región lumbar baja, una o ambas piernas). Puede ser traumática.

Neuralgia del trigémino: síndrome de dolor paroxístico repetitivo en el territorio del trigémino o una o más de sus ramas. Raramente traumática.

Myélopathie post-traumatique : troubles médullaires consécutifs à un traumatisme, chroniques et parfois évolutifs.

Syndrome cervical post-traumatique : voir ce terme.

Anastomose nerveuse : voir *neurorraphie*.

Incarcération nerveuse : voir *incarcération*.

Greffe nerveuse : voir ce terme.

Innervation compensatrice : compensation partielle du déficit dans le territoire d'un nerf périphérique par l'innervation adjacente en cas de section ou compression de ce nerf. La compensation peut être sensitive ou motrice.

Greffe nerveuse : voir ce terme.

Névralgie occipitale : voir *syndrome cervical post-traumatique*.

Névralgie sciatique : algie dans le territoire de distribution sensitive du nerf sciatique (de l'un ou des deux membres inférieurs). L'algie peut être d'origine traumatique.

Névralgie du trijumeau : algie paroxystique récidivante dans le territoire de distribution sensitive du nerf trijumeau ou dans celui d'une ou deux de ses branches. Cette névralgie est rarement d'origine traumatique.

Neurapraxia: see *neuropraxia*.

Neuritis, occipital (suboccipital): see *syndrome*, neck, post-traumatic.

Neuritis, sciatic: usually pain and neurological deficit (sensory and/or motor) in the distribution of sciatic nerve.

Neuritis, tardy ulnar: ulnar nerve dysfunction due to scar, tear or arthritic changes in the epicondylar groove, stretching of nerve from these causes or valgus deformity of the elbow.

Neuroma: 1. a nerve tumor resulting from improper and wild regeneration after a section; when in continuity the neuroma involves the area of damage, when completely sectioned neuroma may develop at the proximal end and a smaller one may develop at the distal end; 2. improper term used for neoplasms arising from nerve cells and fibers such as ganglioneuromas, neurilemmomas, angioneuromas, and others.

Neurapraxie: siehe *neuropraxia* und auch *axonotmesis* und *neurotmesis*.

Okzipital (Subokzipital-) Neuralgie: siehe *syndrome*, neck, posttraumatic.

Ischiassyndrom: Schmerzen und neurologische Ausfälle (sensibel und/oder motorisch) im Ausbreitungsgebiet des Nervus ischiadicus.

Ulnaris-Spätlähmung: Funktionsstörung des Nervus ulnaris infolge Narbe, Dehnung oder arthritischer Veränderungen im Sulcus Nervus ulnaris oder durch Valgus-Stellung des Ellenbogengelenkes, woraus eine Zugschädigung resultiert.

Neurom: 1. knotenförmige Nervenverdickung infolge ungeordnetem Regenerationsvorgang nach Nervenschädigung; bei erhaltener Kontinuität entsteht es in der Schädigungszone, bei völliger Nervendurchtrennung entwickelt es sich am proximalen, geringer am distalen Stumpfende; 2. ungenauer (im Deutschen in diesem Zusammenhang nicht mehr gebräuchlicher) Ausdruck für blastomatöse Veränderungen aus Nervenzellen, die Neurinome.

Neuropraxie : voir ce terme.

Neuritis, occipital (suboccipital): ver *síndrome* cervical post-traumático.

Névrite occipitale : voir *névralgie occipitale.*

Neuritis ciática: generalmente dolor y deficit neurológico sensitivo y/o motor en la distribución del nervio ciático.

Névrite sciatique : déficit neurologique sensitif et/ou moteur et souvent algie dans le territoire du nerf sciatique.

Neuritis cubital tardía: disfunción del nervio cubital por cicatriz, desgarramiento o alteración reumática de la canaleta epicondílea con estiramiento o alteración del nervio por tal causa o por deformación en valgus del codo.

Névralgie, névrite cubitale : troubles neurologiques dans le territoire du nerf cubital du fait d'une cicatrice ou de perturbations d'ordre arthrosique au niveau du canal épicondylien avec étirement du nerf à ce niveau consécutif à ces causes ou à une déformation du coude en valgus.

Neuroma: 1. Tumoración que resulta de la desordenada y exagerada regeneración de un nervio seccionado. El neuroma, cuando es en continuidad, engloba el área lesionado. Cuando la sección es completa puede desarollarse un neuromo en el cabo proximal y otro, más pequeño, en el extremo distal. 2. Término no apropiado que se usa para denominar tumores originados en células o fibras del sistema nervioso: ganglioneuroma, angioneuroma, etc.

Névrome : 1. Cicatrice hypertrophique pseudotumorale développée au niveau d'un nerf périphérique sectionné. Quand il n'y a pas de solution de continuité du nerf, le névrome intéresse la zone lésionnelle. Quand il y a une section totale le névrome peut se développer au niveau de l'extrémité proximale. Un névrome plus petit peut se développer au niveau de l'extrémité distale. 2. Terme improprement utilisé pour désigner des tumeurs vraies des nerfs de la lignée cellulaire ou gliale tels que les ganglioneuromes, les neurinomes, les angioneuromes et autres tumeurs.

Neuropraxia (neurapraxia): loss of axonal conduction but no lesion of the nerve sheaths and no rupture of the axons (Grade I) (see also *axonotmesis* and *neurotmesis*).

Neuropraxie: Nervenverletzung Grad I nur mit Verlust der Axon-Leitfähigkeit, aber ohne Verletzung der Nervenscheiden und ohne Unterbrechung der Axone (siehe auch *axonotmesis*, *neurotmesis*).

Neuropsychiatric disorders, post-traumatic: manifestations due to trauma. May be neurotic, psychotic, behavioral, mental, emotional. May be acute or chronic (see also *encephalopathy, traumatic, chronic* or *syndrome, post-traumatic*).

Psychopathologische Syndrome, posttraumtische: seelische und geistige Störungen nach Hirntrauma. Die englischen und deutschen Sprachinhalte der Begriffe decken sich nicht (siehe *personality disorders*).

Neurorraphy: joining together usually by suture of a divided nerve.

Nervenvereinigung, gewöhnlich durch Naht, bei Nervendurchtrennung.

Neurotmesis: anatomic section of the total nerve sheath and trunk with loss of conduction (Grade III) (see also *neuropraxia* and *axonotmesis*).

Neurotmesis: Nervenschädigung Grad III mit vollständiger Durchtrennung und Funktionsverlust des Nervs (siehe auch *neuropraxia* und *axonotmesis*).

Occlusion, vascular, traumatic: due to extraintimal hemorrhage and/or thrombus after neck and/or head injury.

Gefäßverschluß, traumatischer: infolge Blutung unter die Intima und/oder Thrombose, nach Hals- und/oder Schädeltrauma.

Otorrhea post-traumatic: discharge of CSF, blood or macerated brain from the ear.

Otogene Liquorfistel, posttraumatische: Austritt von (blutigem) Liquor und/oder Hirnbrei aus dem Ohr bei laterobasaler Fraktur.

Neuropraxia: pérdida de la conducción axonal sin ruptura de los axones y sin lesión de las vainas nerviosas (grado I). Ver también *axonotmesis y neurotmesis.*

Neuropraxie : perte de la conduction axonique sans lésion des enveloppes du nerf ni rupture des axones (stade I) (voir aussi *axonotmesis* et *neurotmesis*).

Trastornos neuropsiquiátricos, post-traumáticos: alteraciones debidas al trauma. Pueden ser neuróticas, psicóticas, de comportamiento, mentales, emocionales. Pueden ser agudas o crónicas (ver también *encefalopatía traumática crónica,* o sindrome cerebral crónico traumático).

Troubles psychiques post-traumatiques : les perturbations peuvent être d'ordres neurotique, psychotique, comportemental, mental. Elles peuvent être aigues ou chroniques (voir aussi *encéphalopathie chronique post-traumatique et syndrome subjectif post-traumatique*).

Neurorrafia: unión, generalmente por sutura, de un nervio seccionado.

Neurorraphie : réunion, généralement par suture, des extrémités d'un nerf rompu.

Neurotmesis: sección total del nervio y sus vaina con pérdida de la conducción (grado III) (ver también *neuropraxia y axonotmesis*).

Neurotmésis : section anatomique de la totalité du nerf avec perte de la conduction (stade III) (voir aussi *neuropraxie* et *axonotmesis*).

Obstrucción vascular traumática: debida a hemorragia por fuera de la íntima y/o trombosis luego de traumatismo de cuello y/o cabeza.

Oblitération vasculaire post-traumatique : due à une hémorragie autour de l'intima et/ou une thrombose après un traumatisme cervical et/ou crânien.

Otorrea post-traumática: pérdida de sangre, de líquido cefalorraquídeo, o de substancia cerebral por el oído.

Otorrhée post-traumatique: écoulement de sang, de l. c. r. (oto-liquorrhée) et/ou de matière cérébrale macérée par l'oreille.

Paralysis, compression, nerve: nerve palsy due to prolonged pressure from varying causes such as abnormal prolonged position of an extremity.

Nervendrucklähmung: infolge langer Druckwirkung verschiedener Ursachen, wie langer abnormer Lage einer Extremität.

Personality disorder, post-traumatic: see *neuropsychiatric disorders*, post-traumatic.

Organische Wesensänderung, posttraumatische: geistig-seelische Störung verschiedener Ausprägung, wie Reizbarkeit, Antriebsmangel, Umständlichkeit, Stimmungsschwankung. Die posttraumatisch reversiblen Verläufe werden im Deutschen als Durchgangssyndrom (Wieck 1956) bezeichnet.

Pneumocele (pneumatocele), extracranial (subgaleal emphysema): collection of gas beneath the galea aponeurotica, usually due to fracture into the paranasal sinuses.

Subgaleales Emphysem: Luftansammlung in der Kopfschwarte, gewöhnlich infolge Nasennebenhöhlen-Frakturen.

Pneumocele (pneumatocele), intracranial: collection of gas within the cranial cavity (pneumocephalus) usually due to fracture into the paranasal sinuses or petrous bone. The gas may accumulate within the subdural or subarachnoid spaces, the brain tissue, or the ventricles.

Pneumatozele, intrakranielle: Luftansammlung im Schädelinneren infolge von Frakturen der hirnnahen Wandungen der Nasennebenhöhlen oder des Felsenbeines, im Subdural- oder Subarachnoidalraum, im Gehirngewebe oder in den Ventrikeln (Pneumocephalus).

Post-traumatic syndrome: see *syndrome*, post-traumatic.

Posttraumatisches Syndrom: siehe *syndrome*, post-traumatic.

Parálisis por compresión de un nervio: parálisis por prolongada posición anormal de un nervio.

Paralysie nerveuse par compression : paralysie d'un nerf consécutive à une compression de cause variée, par exemple le maintien d'une position anormale d'une extrémité pendant trop longtemps.

Alteraciones de la personalidad: ver *alteraciones neuropsiquiátricas post-traumáticas.*

Troubles de la personnalité, post-traumatiques : voir *troubles psychiques post-traumatiques.*

Neumocele (neumatocele) extra-craneano (enfisema subgaleal): colección de aire bajo la galea aponeurótica, generalmente por fractura de senos paranasales.

Pneumatocèle (pneumocèle) extra-crânien : collection aérienne sous la galéa, généralement consécutive à une fracture intéressant les sinus périnasaux.

Neumocele (neumatocele) intra-craneano: colección aérea en la cavidad craneana (neumocéfalo) generalmente por fractura de los senos paranasales o del peñasco. El aire puede acumularse en los espacios subdural o subaracnoideo, en el tejido cerebral o en los ventrículos.

Pneumatocèle (pneumocèle) intra-crânien : collection aérienne à l'intérieur de la cavité crânienne (pneumocéphale) généralement due à une fracture des sinus périnasaux ou de l'os pétreux. L'air peut s'accumuler dans l'espace sous-dural, dans les espaces sous-arachnoïdiens, le tissu cérébral ou les ventricules.

ver: *síndrome* post-traumático.

Syndrome subjectif post-traumatique : voir ce terme.

Punch-drunk syndrome: see *syndrome*, punch-drunk.

Schnapstrinker-Syndrom: siehe *syndrome*, punch-drunk.

Rhinorrhea, post-traumatic, cerebrospinal fluid: discharge of cerebrospinal fluid from the nares.

Nasale Liquorfistel, posttraumatische: Abfluß von Hirnflüssigkeit aus der Nase.

Ruptured disk: see *disk*, ruptured.

Perforierter Bandscheibenvorfall: siehe *disk*, ruptured.

Scar, meningocerebral: see *cicatrix*, meningocerebral.

Hirn-Duranarbe: siehe *cicatrix*, meningocerebral.

Sciatica: pain radiating into all or part of the posterior or lateral aspect of the lower limb.

Ischialgie: Schmerzausstrahlung ganz oder teilweise in den hinteren oder lateralen Anteil des Beines.

Sciatic neuralgia: see *neuralgia*, sciatic.

Ischialgie: siehe *neuralgia*, sciatic.

Sciatic neuritis: see *neuritis*, sciatic.

Ischias: siehe *neuritis*, sciatic.

Seizures, immediate, post-traumatic: seizures occuring in the first few days after a brain trauma. Usually do not imply epilepsy (see also *epilepsy*, post-traumatic).

Anfälle, frühe, posttraumatische: hirnorganische Anfälle während der ersten Tage nach Hirntraumen, gewöhnlich nicht in rezidivierende Anfälle — Anfallsleiden — übergehend (siehe auch *epilepsy*, post-traumatic).

Skull fracture, closed-open: see *skull fracture*, closed-open in *craniocerebral injury*.

Schädelfraktur, geschlossene, offene: siehe *skull fracture*, closed-open in *craniocerebral injury*.

ver: *síndrome* de borrachera por golpes.

Encéphalopathie des boxeurs : troubles neuro-psychiques chroniques dûs à des traumatismes cranio-cérébraux répétés (en boxe) et caractérisés par une détérioration émotionnelle et/ou mentale et/ou des déficits moteurs.

Craneo-rinorrea, post-traumática: pérdida de L. C. R. por la nariz.

Rhinorrhée cérébro-spinale post-traumatique : écoulement de l. c. r. par les narines.

ver: *disco* intervertebral roto.

Rupture discale : voir ce terme.

ver: *cicatriz* meningocerebral.

Cicatrice cérébro-méningée : voir ce terme.

Ciática: dolor irradiado o todo o a parte de un miembro inferior, por su lado externo o posterior.

Sciatique : algie irradiant au niveau de la face postérieure d'un membre inférieur en partie ou en totalité.

ver: *neuralgia* ciática.

Névralgie sciatique : voir ce terme.

ver: *neuritis* ciática.

Névrite sciatique : voir ce terme.

Ataques (convulsiones) post-traumáticos inmediatos: ataques que ocurren en los primeros días consecutivos a un trauma. Generalmente no indican epilepsia (ver también *epilepsia* post-traumática).

Crises épileptiques dans les suites immédiates d'un traumatisme : crises épileptiques survenant dans les premiers jours qui suivent un traumatisme cérébral. Généralement elles ne signifient pas l'apparition d'une épilepsie post-traumatique (voir aussi *épilepsie post-traumatique*).

ver: *fractura* de cráneo cerrada-abierta, en *traumatismo* encéfalo-craneano.

Fracture fermée, ouverte du crâne : voir ce terme dans la rubrique *traumatismes cranio-cérébraux*.

4*

Splint: a device to immobilize and prevent motion of a body part (see also *brace*).

Spondylolisthesis: generally anterior displacement of the body of a vertebra on the one below, usually the fifth lumbar vertebra on the sacrum. In some cases, doubtful traumatic etiology.

Sprain, vertebral (cervical-dorsal-lumbosacral): injury with stretching, tearing or rupture of some ligaments and muscles. No dislocation or fracture.

Sprain fracture, vertebral (cervical-dorsal-lumbosacral): stress resulting in a small portion of bone being pulled or pushed off. "Tear Drop" fracture, fracture of the transverse process and of spinous process are examples.

Strain, vertebral (cervical-dorsal-lumbosacral): stretching of ligaments, tendons, and muscles with neckache or backache lasting a short time.

Subdural, hematoma: see *hematoma*.

Subluxation, vertebral: an incomplete dislocation with articular surfaces in partial contact. There is a loss of normal relationship.

Schiene: Vorrichtung zur Ruhigstellung eines Körperteils (siehe auch *brace* = Halter, Stützkorsett).

Spondylolisthesis, Wirbelgleiten: Abgleiten eines Wirbels, meistens nach vorne, auf dem darunterliegenden Wirbel, gewöhnlich 5. Lenden- gegenüber 1. Kreuzbeinwirbel. In einigen Fällen fraglich traumatischer Ätiologie.

Verrenkung, Distorsion der Hals-, Brust-, Lendenwirbelsäule: Unfall mit Zerrung, Dehnung oder Ruptur von Bändern und Muskeln. Keine Dislokation oder Fraktur.

Verrenkungsbruch der Hals-, Brust-, Lendenwirbelsäule: Gewalteinwirkung mit Abriß oder Abscherung eines kleinen Knochenstückes, wie Wirbelkörperrandkanten-Absprengung, Querfortsatz- oder Dornfortsatz-Bruch.

Zerrung der Hals-, Brust-, Lendenwirbelsäule: Überdehnung von Bändern, Sehnen und Muskeln mit kurzdauernden Nacken- oder Rückenschmerzen.

Subdurales Hämatom: siehe *hematoma*.

Subluxation, Wirbel-: unvollständige Verlagerung, bei welcher die Wirbelgelenkflächen in Teilkontakt bleiben, aber der normale anatomische Bezug verloren geht.

53

Ortesis: dispositivo para inmovilizar un segmento corporal.

Corset, minerve : voir ces termes.

Espondilolistesis: desplazamiento, por la común hacia adelante, del cuerpo de una vértebra sobre el de la inmediamente inferior, generalmente la quinta sobre el sacro. En algunos casos es de etiología traumática dudosa.

Spondylolisthésis : Glissement, généralement en avant, d'un corps vertébral par rapport au sousjacent, fréquemment la 5ème vertèbre lombaire par rapport au sacrum. Dans quelques cas une étiologie traumatique peut être évoquée.

Esguince vertebral (cervical-dorsal-lumbo-sacro): lesión con estiramiento, desgarradura o rotura de algunos ligamentos y músculos. No hay dislocación ni fractura.

Entorse vertébrale : traumatisme avec étirement, déchirure ou rupture de quelques ligaments et muscles. Il n'y a ni luxation ni fracture.

Fractura por arrancamiento: como resultado de la tensión se desprende un fragmento de hueso. Ejemplos: las fracturas „en gota" y las fracturas de las apófisis transversas o espinosas.

Entorse grave (fractures parcellaires) : un fragment osseux vertébral a été fracturé par pulsion ou arrachement. Les fractures en larme, les fractures des apophyses transverses ou des apophyses épineuses en sont des exemples.

Distensión vertebral: estiramiento de ligamentos, tendones y músculos con dolor cervical o dorsolumbar de corta duración.

Lumbago, torticolis : étirement des ligaments, des tendons ou des muscles avec algies lombaires ou cervicales d'une durée limitée.

ver: *hematoma.*

Hématome sous-dural : voir ce terme dans la rubrique *hematomes intracrâniens.*

Subluxacion vertebral: dislocación incompleta, manteniendo las apófisis articulares un contacto parcial. Hay pérdida de la relación normal.

Subluxation rachidienne : luxation incomplète avec contact des articulaires partiellement conservé. Il n'y a pas de perturbations importantes des rapports anatomiques normaux.

Sudeck's atrophy: neurovascular syndrome due to trauma of extremity characterized by spotty decalcification of bone or bones with severe pain in the extremity. Early there may be swelling, vasodilation and cyanosis. Later there may be pallor and glossy skin.

Sudeck-Atrophie: neurovasculäres Syndrom nach Extremitätenverletzung, charakterisiert durch fleckige Knochenentkalkung und starke Schmerzen. Im akuten Stadium können Schwellung, Vasodilatation und Cyanose bestehen, in späteren Stadien jedoch Blässe und Glanzhaut.

Swelling, brain-spinal cord: a pathological entity characterized by an increase in bulk of nervous tissue, due to expansion of the intravascular (*congestion*) or extravascular (edema) compartments. These may coexist or may occur separately and be clinically indistinguishable. The process may be limited or diffuse.

Hirn-Schwellung, Rückenmarks-: eine pathologische Einheit, charakterisiert durch eine Volumenzunahme des Hirn- oder Rückenmarkgewebes infolge Ausdehnung des intravaskulären (Stauung) oder extravaskulären (Ödem) Gewebsanteiles. Diese Formen können miteinander bestehen oder getrennt auftreten und klinisch nicht unterscheidbar sein. Der Prozeß kann umschrieben oder diffus sein.

Syndrome, acute anterior cervical cord: an incomplete lesion with immediate paralysis of the four extremities with loss of pain and temperature and preservation of posterior column function. Sphincter paralysis.

Spinalis-Anterior-Syndrom, akutes: eine unvollständige Halsmarkschädigung mit akuter Tetraparese und dissoziierten Empfindungsstörungen, Blasen- und Mastdarmlähmung.

Atrofia de Sudeck: síndrome neurovascular debido a trauma de un miembro y que se caracteriza por decalcificación irregular de uno o más huesos e intenso dolor de la extremidad. En un primer periodo puede haber edema, vasodilatación y cianósis. Más tarde puede haber palidez y piel brillosa.

Syndrome atrophique de Sudeck : syndrome neurovasculaire consécutif à un traumatisme d'une extrémité caractérisé par une décalcification « mouchetée » d'un ou plusieurs os avec importante algie distale. Il peut s'installer précocement un oedème, une vasodilatation et une cyanose. Ultérieurement les téguments peuvent être pâles et brillants.

Edema, cerebral-medular: entidad patológica caracterizada por un aumento del volumen del tejido nervioso debido a, o expansión del compartimiento vascular (congestión) o del compartimiento extravascular (edema verdadero). Ambos pueden coexistir u ocurrir por separado y ser clinicamente indiferenciables. El proceso puede ser limitado o difuso.

Oedème cérébral, médullaire : état pathologique cérébral caractérisé par une augmentation de volume du tissu nerveux due à une expansion du secteur intravasculaire (congestion) ou extravasculaire (oedème vrai). Les deux peuvent se superposer ou apparaître séparément sans qu'il soit possible de faire une distinction clinique. Le processus peut être limité ou diffus.

Síndrome agudo, anterior de la médula cervical: lesión incompleta con parálisis inmediata de los cuatro miembros, pérdida de sensibilidad al dolor y a la temperatura y preservación de la función de los cordones posteriores. Hay parálisis esfinteriana.

Syndrome antéro-médullaire cervical aigu : lésion médullaire cervicale partielle avec paralysie immédiate des 4 membres, avec abolition de la sensibilité à la douleur et à la température et conservation des fonctions des cordons postérieurs. Paralysie sphinctérienne.

Syndrome, acute central cervical cord: an incomplete lesion with severe loss of motor function of upper extremities and partial preservation of motor function of lower extremities; varying sensory losses; sphincter paralysis.

Akute zentrale Halsmarkschädigung: inkompletter Halsmarkquerschnitt mit schweren Paresen der Arme, aber partiell erhaltener Motorik der Beine sowie verschiedengradigen sensiblen Störungen, Blasen-Mastdarm-Lähmung.

Syndrome, carpal tunnel: tingling, burning and numbness of the hand (acroparesthesia) in the distribution of the median nerve resulting from neural compression by the flexor retinaculum.

Karpaltunnel-Syndrom: Prickeln, Brennen und Taubheitsgefühl der Hand im Ausbreitungsgebiet des Nervus medianus infolge Kompression dieses Nervs unter dem Retinaculum flexorum im Canalis carpi.

Syndrome, cervical, tension: see *syndrome*, neck, post-traumatic.

Nackensteife: siehe *syndrome*, neck, post-traumatic.

Syndrome, neck, post-traumatic (occipital or suboccipital neuralgia or neuritis, tension headache, cervical tension syndrome, cervical myospasm): a clinical complex of pain tenderness, stiff neck, muscle spasm, vasomotor instability and ill-defined symptoms as dizziness, blurred vision, etc.

Zervikalsyndrom, posttraumatisches: ein klinischer Komplex von Schmerz, Empfindlichkeit, Spasmus der Nackenmuskulatur und vasomotorischen Störungen, wie Taumeligkeit, Verschwommensehen.

Syndrome, postconcussion: see *syndrome*, post-traumatic.

Postcontusionelles Syndrom: siehe *syndrome*, post-traumatic.

Syndrome, post-traumatic: a clinical complex characterized by headache, dizziness, neurasthenia, hypersensitivity to stimuli and diminished concentration.

Posttraumatisches Syndrom: ein klinischer Komplex, charakterisiert durch Kopfschmerzen, Schwindel, vorzeitige Erschöpfung, Reizbarkeit und Konzentrationsschwäche.

Síndrome agudo, central de la médula cervical: lesión incompleta con severa pérdida de motilidad en los miembros superiores y preservación motora parcial en las extremidades inferiores. Hay alteraciones sensitivas de grado variable y parálisis esfinteriana.

Síndrome del tunel carpiano: hormigueo, sensación quemante y adormecimiento de la mano (acroparestesias) en el territorio del nervio mediano por compresión de éste por el ligamento anterior del carpo.

Síndrome de tensión cervical: ver *síndrome* cervical post-traumático.

Síndrome cervical post-traumático (neuralgia o neuritis occipital o suboccipital, cefalea de tensión, síndrome de tensión cervical, mioespasmo cervical): complejo clínico de dolor, hiperalgesia, espasmo de músculos cervicales, inestabilidad vasomotor a y síntomas mal definidos como mareo, visión borrosa, etc.

Síndrome post-conmocional: ver *síndrome* post-traumático.

Síndrome post-traumático: complejo clínico caracterizado por cefalea, mareo, neurastenia, hipersensibilidad a los estímulos y pobre concentración mental.

Syndrome centro-médullaire cervical aigu : lésion médullaire cervicale partielle avec importante diminution de la motricité des membres supérieurs et préservation partielle de celle des membres inférieurs. Déficits sensitifs variables. Paralysie sphinctérienne.

Syndrome du canal carpien : fourmillements, brûlures et engourdissement de la main (acroparesthésies) dans le territoire de distribution du nerf médian consécutifs à la compression du nerf dans le canal.

Syndrome cervical post-traumatique : voir ce terme.

Syndrome cervical post-traumatique : ensemble complexe de douleurs, de sensibilité exacerbée, de contracture des muscles cervicaux, d'instabilité vasomotrice et de symptômes mal définis tels que sensations vertigineuses, vision trouble.

Syndrome subjectif post-commotionnel : voir *syndrome subjectif post-traumatique.*

Syndrome subjectif post-traumatique : ensemble complexe de troubles avec des céphalées, des sensations vertigineuses, une tendance à l'anxiété, une hypersensibilité aux différents stimuli, une difficulté de concentration intellectuelle.

58

Syndrome, punch-drunk: a form of a chronic neuropsychiatric disorder due to repeated head trauma (in boxing) characterized by emotional and/or mental impairment and/or motor deficit.

Syndrome, traumatic chronic brain: see *encephalopathy*, traumatic chronic (see also *neuropsychiatric disorders*, post-traumatic).

"Tear drop" fracture: see *fracture*, "tear drop".

Tear, vascular: tear of artery and/or vein with varying degrees of hemorrhage depending on the size of the vessel, may form dissecting or false aneurysm.

Tension headache: see *syndrome*, neck, post-traumatic.

Thrombosis, post-traumatic (arterial or venous): intravascular clotting due to injury to a vessel wall.

Tomography: radiographic imaging of body sections.

Tomography, computerized (C.T.): computerized analysis of tomographic densities.

Schnaps-Trinker-Syndrom: eine Form chronischer neurologisch-psychischer Veränderungen infolge wiederholter Hirntraumen (wie Boxen), bestehend aus Gefühls- und/oder Gedächtnisstörungen und/oder neurologischen Ausfällen.

Traumatische Hirndauerschädigung: siehe auch *neuropsychiatric disorders*, post-traumatic; siehe *encephalopathy*, traumatic chronic.

Tränen-Tropfen-Fraktur: siehe *fracture*, „tear drop".

Gefäßzerrung: Dehnung einer Arterie und/oder Vene mit verschieden starker Blutung in Abhängigkeit vom Gefäßkaliber oder mit Bildung eines Aneurysma dissecans oder eines Aneurysma spurium.

Kopfschmerz: verbunden mit reflektorischer Muskelverspannung, Nervosität, Ängstlichkeit; siehe *syndrome*, neck, post-traumatic.

Thrombose, posttraumatische (arterielle oder venöse): intravaskuläre Blutgerinnung infolge traumatischer Schädigung der Gefäßwand.

Tomographie: Röntgenschichtbild.

Computer-Tomographie: computerausgewertete Röntgenschichtuntersuchung intrakorporaler Dichteunterschiede.

Síndrome de borrachera por golpes: forma de alteración neuropsiquiátrica crónica secundaria a traumas cefálicos repetidos (en el boxeo) y que se caracteriza por deterioro emocional y/o mental y/o déficit motor.

Encéphalopathie des boxeurs : voir ce terme.

Síndrome cerebral crónico posttraumático: ver *encefalopatía* crónica traumática.

Encéphalopathie chronique posttraumatique : voir ce terme (voir aussi *troubles psychiques posttraumatiques*).

Tear drop „fracture": ver *fractura* „en gota".

Fracture en larme : voir ce terme.

Ruptura vascular: ruptura de una arteria y/o vena con grado variable de hemorragia según el tamaño del vaso. Puede originar un aneurisma disecante o falso aneurisma.

Plaie vasculaire : voir ce terme.

Cefalea por tensión: ver *síndrome* cervical post-traumático.

Syndrome cervical post-traumatique : voir ce terme.

Trombosis, post-traumática (arterial o venosa): coagulación intravascular debida a lesión de la pared del vaso.

Thrombose artérielle ou veineuse post-traumatique : thrombus intravasculaire se constituant du fait du traumatisme.

Tomografía: imágen radiográfica de planos corporales.

Tomographie : images radiographiques en section du corps.

Tomografía computada (T. C.): representación planigráfica del análisis computado de densidades tomográficas.

Tomographie computérisée (T. C.): représentation planigraphique de l'analyse par ordinateur des densités tomographiques (densitométrie, tacographie).

Tonsillar herniation: see *herniation,* foraminal (tonsillar).

Traction, cervical: mechanical device providing a constant pull on the head and neck to overcome muscular spasm and realign the cervical spine. Traction with Crutchfield Tongs, Halter traction, etc.

Traction, halter: traction of head and neck with chin sling connected to a weight over a pulley (see also *chin sling*).

Traction, pelvic: mechanical device provided to produce traction on the pelvis to overcome muscular spasm and produce normal realignment of vertebrae.

Uncal herniation: see *herniation,* transtentorial, caudal.

Uncounsciousness, traumatic: total loss of perception of environment and self.

Vascular occlusion: see *occlusion,* vascular.

Vascular tear: see *tear,* vascular.

Tonsillen-Einklemmung: siehe *herniation,* foraminal (tonsillar).

Extension der Halswirbelsäule: Vorrichtung zur Ausübung eines konstanten Zuges an Kopf und Nacken zur Überwindung des Muskelspasmus und Wiederaufrichtung der Halswirbelsäule, z. B. Crutchfield-Zange, Glisson-Schlinge.

Halter-Schlinge: Kopf- und Nackenzug mit Kinnschleuder, die über eine Rolle mit einem Gewicht verbunden ist (siehe auch *chin sling*).

Becken-Zug: Zugvorrichtung am Becken zur Überwindung des Muskelspasmus und zur Wiederaufrichtung der Wirbelsäule.

Uncus-Prolaps, Temporallappen-Hernie, Tentoriumschlitz-Einklemmung: siehe auch *herniation,* transtentorial, caudal.

Bewußtlosigkeit, posttraumatische: Fehlen geistiger Wahrnehmung der Umgebung und seiner selbst.

Gefäßverschluß: siehe *occlusion,* vascular.

Gefäßzerrung: siehe *tear,* vascular.

Hernia amigdalina: ver *hernia* foraminal o amigdalina.

Tracción cervical: dispositivo mecánico que permite una tracción permanente de la cabeza y cuello para contrarrestar el espasmo muscular y permitir realinear la columna cervical. Tracción con pinza de Crutchfield, tracción con fronda, etc.

Tracción con fronda: tracción de cabeza y cuello por una fronda mentoniana conectada a un peso sobre una polea.

Tracción pelviana: dispositivo mecánico para traccionar la pelvis, contrarrestar el espasmo muscular, y permitir realinear normalmente las vértebras.

Hernia del uncus: ver *hernia* transtentorial descendente.

Inconciencia: pérdida total de la percepción del medio y de si mismo.

ver: *oclusión* vascular.

ver: *ruptura* vascular.

Engagement amygdalien : voir *hernie amygdalienne.*

Traction cervicale : appareillage réalisant une traction constante sur l'extrémité céphalique et le cou pour lutter contre la contracture musculaire et réduire les troubles statiques de la colonne cervicale. Traction avec broche de Crutchfield, fronde etc.

Traction cervicale par fronde : traction de la tête et du cou à l'aide d'une fronde reliée par une poulie à un contre-poids.

Traction pelvienne : appareillage réalisant une traction sur le pelvis pour lutter contre la contracture musculaire et réduire les troubles statiques vertébraux.

Engagement de l'uncus temporal : voir *hernie temporale.*

Inconscience post-traumatique : perte totale de la perception de l'environnement et de soi-même.

Oblitération vasculaire : voir ce terme.

Plaie vasculaire : plaie d'une artère ou d'une veine avec degré varié d'hémorragie selon le calibre du vaisseau et susceptible de donner naissance à une dissection vasculaire ou à un faux anévrysme.

Vertigo: a sensation of rotation or displacement relative to environment.

Schwindel: Gefühl der Drehung oder unwillkürlichen Bewegung gegenüber der Umgebung.

Whiplash injury: see *injury*, whiplash.

Schleudertrauma: Peitschenhiebverletzung (siehe *injury*, whiplash).

Wound, penetrating, craniocerebral: open wound in which the dura mater is pierced.

Offene Schädel-Hirn-Verletzung: Verletzung der Weichteile, des Knochens und der darunterliegenden Dura.

Wound, penetrating, spine: open wound into the spinal canal with piercing of the dura mater.

Offene Rückenmarksverletzung: bis in den Wirbelkanal reichende Verletzung mit Eröffnung der Dura.

Wound, perforating, craniocerebral: a wound which traverses the cranial cavity and the integument.

Schädelverletzung, transversale (z. B. Schädeldurchschuß): durchquert den Schädel und seine Hüllen.

Wound, perforating, spine: wound traversing the spine and the skin.

Wirbelsäulenverletzung, transversale: Verletzung, die die Wirbelsäule und ihre Hüllen durchquert.

Wound, puncture: laceration in which the orifice is relatively small compared to the depth.

Pfählungsverletzung: Verletzung mit relativ kleiner Eintrittsöffnung im Vergleich zu ihrer Tiefe.

Wound, tangential, skull-spine ("gutter", "crease"): a wound made by a missile the trajectory of which is tangential to the curvature of the skull or to the spine.

Tangential-Schuß, Schädel-/Wirbelsäule (Rinnen-Schuß): der Schußkanal streift tangentenartig die Schädelwölbung bzw. Wirbelsäule.

Vértigo: sensación de rotación o de desplazamiento en relación al medio.

ver: *traumatismo cervical* en „*latigazo*".

Herida penetrante craneocerebral: herida abierta con perforación de duramadre.

Herida penetrante, raquídea: herida abierta del raquis con apertura de duramadre.

Herida perforante craneocerebral: herida penetrante que atraviesa la caja craneana y los tegumentos.

Herida perforante, raquídea: herida que atraviesa la columna y los tegumentos.

Herida puntiforme: laceración en la cual el orificio de entrada es comparativamente pequeño en relación a su profundidad.

Herida tangencial „en canaleta" de cráneo o columna: herida hecha por un proyectil cuya trayectoria es tangencial a la curvatura del cráneo o de la columna.

Vertiges : sensation de rotation ou de déplacement.

Coup de fouet cervical, coup de fléau cervical : voir ce terme.

Plaie craniocérébrale : plaie des enveloppes crâniennes, dure-mère comprise.

Plaie rachidienne : plaie des tissus de recouvrement rachidien et de la dure-mère.

Plaie perforante cranio-cérébrale en séton : plaie traversant de part en part le crâne et les téguments.

Plaie perforante rachidienne : plaie traversant les tissus de recouvrement rachidien et le rachis de part en part.

Plaie punctiforme : plaie dont l'orifice est étroit, mais qui est susceptible d'être profonde.

Plaie tangentielle du crâne, du rachis : plaie par projectile dont la trajectoire est tangentielle au crâne ou au rachis.